"In a time of universal decei *truth as steadfastly as he pr(*

Becky Akers

"I love Allan's writings on HOW TO avoid wearing the fear mask. Practical information as well as resistance theory."

Bo Andersen

"I first came across the writings of my friend Allan Stevo when I read this book of his:

How to Win America for Ron Paul and the Cause of Freedom in 2012;

I was gratified by the fact that his book ran very strongly parallel to my own, on the same topic:

Yes to Ron Paul and Liberty.

My only 'problem' with that book of his was that I had wished I had included in my own book many of the things he wrote in his.

Ever since then, I have been an avid reader, and fan, of Allan's. He is a regular contributor to LewRockwell.com (as am I), and again, I have found him to be a kindred spirit, in our mutual effort to promote liberty. What does his writing mean to me? All the world."

Dr. Walter E. Block

"Public health officials are lying to you. Read this book to get the real skinny on 'chin diapers.' It might be the most important thing you can do for yourself, your family, and your country besides signing the Great Barrington Declaration: https://gbdeclaration.org/."

Professor Robert E. Wright

"Allan Stevo's unbroken work on the topic of masks has given me and countless others useful information to face these strange times fearlessly. Thanks to the advice in Face Masks in One Lesson I was able to safely travel across the country by plane, train, and automobile without a mask or harassment."

Zac Wendroff

"Allan Stevo is a front line warrior in a battle against the Leviathan State and the propagandists for it. His battle against Face Mask Lunacy must be understood and appreciated in that context."

Mark Dankof

"Allan Stevo is passionate about promoting effective public policy while discarding dogma, conventional wisdom, and trendy memes. He is relentless in his pursuit of truth and sanity. He is courageous and does not fear the likely public blowback that his unconventional work is likely to elicit."

Mark Abell

"Allan Stevo's new book is one of the myriad thought catalysts that will accelerate US to Veritas = Truth & Reality."

Thaddeus A. Zatori

"Stevo's writing represents a pursuit of the truth with an understanding of our current place in history."

Matt Michael

"Nothing should be forced on our faces or into our bodies 'for the greater good.' This deceitful communist slogan is being used to rob us of our God-given rights. I am grateful for Allan Stevo's book, which is urgently needed in defending this ancient boundary."

Ashkan Jafarpisheh

"Your writings are doses of tranquility for my rage and semi inferno due to the subjectification brought upon my life in recent months."

Hoseyn Vosouq

"Another home run for you. So much sense in your analyses of the multiplicity of mask 'checkpoint' scenarios. It's all about picking battles and adjusting tactics in order to win the war."

Mark Higdon

"Face masks are dog training for medical tyranny — be a 'bad dog' / good human, and read this book!"

Nick Taylor

"You're writing is an asset that provides the people with the educational and informational power to resist the forced mask tyranny. In many Muslim countries, women are oppressed into tyrannically being forced to wear hijabs. Masks are the new hijabs. This tyranny needs to end as soon as it was never supposed to start."

Krishna Chandrasekaran

"Allan Stevo's articles on face masks have provided invaluable information and confidence in my personal efforts to educate people and liberate faces. I am excited to have Allan's knowledge and encouragement at my fingertips with Face Masks in One Lesson. Thank you Allan, keep up the good fight against the face mask illusion."

Karen Stansberry

"It's amazing how people with no scientific background act like medical experts these days. I'm glad we have Allan Stevo to rally opposition to mindless mask fascists."

Michael Denny

"Your words are clear, concise, and an encouragement as you issue condign judgement upon tyranny."

Daniel Bjorndahl

"Many books will tell you what to do but not how to do it. This is not one of those books! Mr. Stevo tells you exactly what to find out, what to say, and what not to say to maximize your freedom in the era of 'face diapering.'"

Scott Olmsted

"Allan Stevo is one of the rare individuals in our world today that operates under reason, logic and common sense. Place to the side your 'faith' in what the main stream narrative is and after reading the writings of Allan your mind will be challenged to utilize those qualities you were born with. I can hardly wait to read each and every post that Allan does because he WILL challenge your too often than not wrong way of thinking!"

Mark Reynolds

"Mr. Stevo provides humanity a glorious example of respectful & constructive efforts to effect legitimate change. Evident is his concern for personalized health, application of medical research, due process & fighting the good fight against systemic invasions on liberty.

Quitting my occupation due to corporate mask mandates, Mr. Stevo has provided hope that future mask mandates will be resisted peacefully."

Alex Morris

"What a great book!"

Lisa Jackson

"Allan Stevo has shown what logical thinking, a stalwart attitude toward approaching the 'gatekeepers' at the front door, and a sincere desire to eliminate this unnecessary mandate to wear masks can do for you."

Walter Dubyna

"Allan Stevo's entertaining style and insightful linkage of 'fear masks' with government psychological warfare so early in the COVID scamdemic was instrumental in inspiring and informing my own activism on this issue."

John Tieber

"Experts, bureaucrats and politicians don't advise you of your rights when they issue unconstitutional edicts such as face mask orders. You can assert your rights without being or hiring an attorney - it's actually quite easy. Allan Stevo's practical tips show the way, empowering each of us to heed our instincts and find our voice."

Pam Buttram

"You have been a precedence of sanity in a seemingly increasingly unsound world.

When I feel weak and bereft of hope your voice splits the darkness in the nick of time and reminds me I don't have to capitulate to this tyranny."

Jeri Dietz

"Thank you for the truth in print."

Mike Falls

"Allan Stevo is a beacon of liberty. He has inspired my wife and I to push back against the mask madness at every opportunity."

Bill Spitz

"Healthy people should not be wearing masks! That is my professional opinion as a registered nurse. People should NOT be held hostage by unreasonable fear. Thank you, Allan Stevo, for working to stop this disgusting practice."

Joyce Smith, RN

"Far and away the most brilliant and insightful approach to the mask conditioning issue I have seen anywhere ... ever. Its genius in deflection and mitigation of response offers the most valuable tools anyone who has railed against the mask issue has likely even thought about. If we dont stop this trend now ... Where we end up will shock all in its severity. I thank you deeply for this insight!"

Ric Desan

"Allan has an ability to take complicated matters and put them into simple English that the average person can understand. He's not looking to simply educate but also to motivate people to action out of a sense of duty with the liberty with which they have been entrusted."

Tim Brown

"As government mask propaganda intensifies, we very much need the truth. That's why you should read this book."

Llewellyn H. Rockwell, Jr.

Face Masks
In One Lesson

Face Masks
In One Lesson

Allan Stevo

INTRODUCTION

THE LESSON

THE LESSON APPLIED

NUTS AND BOLTS

CONDITIONS

ADVANCED APPLICATIONS OF THE LESSON

CONCLUSION

AFTERWORD

APPENDIX

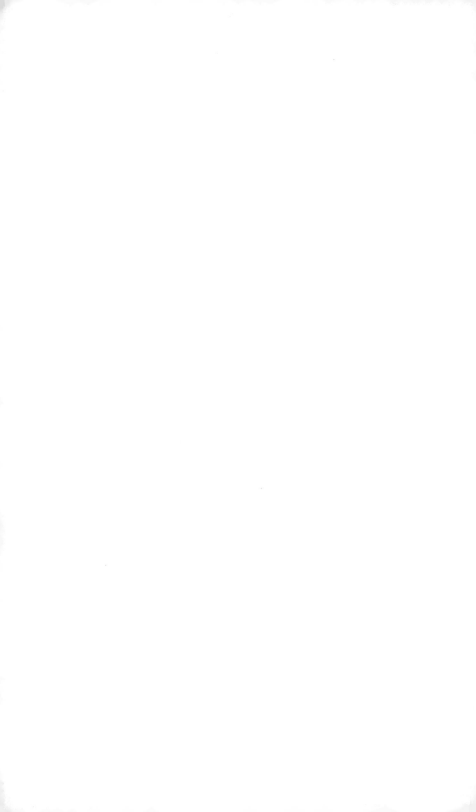

Amaryllidi:

May you be as insightful
as they come
about the words of others.

May you know
no tacit approval,
neither given
nor received.

Introduction

All Advancement Begins With One Decision

A review of the gold standard control randomized trials with laboratory confirmed outcomes published in the May 2020 *Emerging Infectious Disease*, a Center for Disease Control and Prevention (CDC) journal, says unequivocally that face masks don't stop the spread of Covid-19 and should not be relied on to do so.

Here's a quote from the study:

> "Although mechanistic studies support the potential effect of hand hygiene or face masks, evidence from 14 randomized controlled trials of these measures did not support a substantial effect on transmission of laboratory-confirmed influenza. We similarly found limited evidence on the effectiveness of improved hygiene and environmental cleaning. We identified several major knowledge gaps requiring further research, most fundamentally an improved characterization of the modes of person-to-person transmission."

That's right:

1.) It doesn't matter if you sanitize surfaces.
2.) It doesn't matter if you wash your hands.
3.) Masks don't work.

Furthermore, the study says:

Fit Testing — N95 and P2 respirators require proper fit testing to guarantee effectiveness.

Single Use — Used respirators must be immediately disposed of to guarantee effectiveness, neither being reused nor left out.

Hand Contact — To guarantee effectiveness, respirators should not be touched with unwashed hands during use.

Nose and Mouth — The mouth and nose must not be touched during respirator use to guarantee effectiveness.

Hand Hygiene — Hands must be washed every time after touching a used respirator to guarantee effectiveness and only washed hands should be used to touch a sterile respirator.

Moisture Accumulation — Damp masks must be immediately replaced to guarantee effectiveness.

Poorly done studies say face masks may work. Mechanistic studies say the theory behind face masks should work. However, when it comes down to laboratory confirmed evidence, it is clear that face masks don't work to stop the spread of Covid and may actually be harmful. You won't hear that in the news.

In fact, this study entitled "Nonpharmaceutical Measures for Pandemic Influenza in Nonhealthcare Settings – Personal Protective and Environmental

Measures" by Dr. Jingyi Xiao[1] from the University of Hong Kong has effectively been buried.

2020 is the year everyone was masked. You'd think this study would be well received. Instead of being the groundbreaking journal article of 2020 and cited hundreds of times, as of the date of this writing, this journal article, has been only cited 21 times.

A bunch of uninformed Chicken Littles are stressing everyone out by imposing these face masks on society.

The Chicken Littles, unfortunately, have the mouthpiece of the media on their side and in some cases the force of law as well. That doesn't stop them from being so very mistaken. The science is clear. Gold standard studies say the masks don't work.

What's worse, mask orders are being followed by those who might be expected to be reliable bulwarks to such inanity. Some of these bulwarks need rescuing from the toxic idea that has gotten hold of them.

The fable of Chicken Little instructively warns not just to avoid following fear-mongering Chicken Little, but to also avoid the sly foxes who see the situation for what it is and who will happily use it to their advantage.

What is a thinking person to do? Well this book is for you. If you agree that masks aren't for you, this book will help you to never again wear a mask.

The only chapter you need is the first chapter. After reading that I'd say close the book and move on with your life. Please do the world a favor and pass this book along to another, for it is on bookshelves that good ideas grow stale. For slow learners, like me, the rest of the book exists to elaborate on the first chapter – The Lesson — and further drive that point home. I write this book, in the service of you, the thinking man, as we do our best to navigate this world that demands that unchecked emotion take center stage.

Man is not beast. Man has the ability to choose to utilize faculties of reason and to improve himself to become better at recognizing those opportunities and seizing them, lifting himself and those around him from the life of a beast.

This maddening "year," which could last for one year, ten years, or a thousand years, will not be brought to an end by chance, by edict or by unchecked emotion. It will be brought to an end by thinking man doing what thinking man has always done: acting in an individual capacity that results in him pulling himself and others around him up from the mire of unchecked emotion.

How important feelings are. How important reason is. How interfering unchecked emotion can be in creating a better life.

Every moment of life, every instant of life can be better. This is at the foundation of economic thought: human wants are infinite, but resources finite. Progress takes place by man wanting better, despite his limited resources.

Unchecked emotion distracts from that drive. Healthy human feeling and the faculty for reason empower that drive.

The advancement of civilization depends on the individual in every age to make that decision to propel himself forward against the prevailing tide of his era. That prevailing tide so often calls for more of the same, and less of the better.

In this aspect, no era is any different than the era we live in today. Every era requires the individual to choose to make that decision or not. And when that decision is made, it determines the role that individual will play in shaping his own future and the trajectory of his society. It all begins with one decision by one individual and this responsibility is nothing to fret about. It is to be embraced as an important part of how reality functions. Before our religious leaders were all such whiners, this is what a pope had to say about the role of man in life: "Let us thank God that He makes us live among the present problems. It is no longer permitted to anyone to be mediocre."

Yes, one can choose to act in the hallmark of modern American liberalism and ignore reality, because it isn't the reality one wants. Alternately, one can choose to embrace reality and move on with acceptance in addressing the world with renewed vigor and knowledge. The reality is: it's up to you. No era has seen advancement in any other way. In doing so, change is guaranteed to you. You can and will have meaningful impact on the world by resolving to have that impact.

It may be your own life you change: the most certain impact you are guaranteed. You may also surprise yourself by changing a few lives of those around you.

It may not stop there, your individual action, perhaps merely taken out of your own self-interest, may ripple out so much further, in ways immeasurable as bold action has been known to do.

The Roman writer Virgil advised about decisions like that, a decision that faces the individual at every turn in life sometimes many times a day.

In Latin it was "Tu ne cede malis sed contra audentior ito." In English: "Do not give in to evil, but proceed ever more boldly against it."

I invite you to read this first chapter and to go out and live your life knowing that you will change your own life, the life that must be most important to you, and knowing too that the ripples you create may ripple out with immeasurable impact.

Who is with me?

Allan Stevo
September 17, 2020
Carmel-by-the-Sea, California

The Lesson

The Lesson

Three common ways to stop wearing a face mask are as follows:

<u>Method 1</u>: Just stop and don't acknowledge the existence of face masks. Live life normally.

<u>Method 2</u>: Just stop and ask for permission all along the way.

<u>Method 3</u>: Invoke an exemption.

The First Method

The most admirable of these three ways is the first. It presumes one has the personal freedom to make their own medical choices and then lives accordingly.

The only problem is that not everyone is willing to let a free man live like a free man.

Consequently, the first method does not always work well.

The people who can pull it off are amazing and the places where it works are so hospitable to freedom.

It's beautiful to watch and speaks volumes about the individual doing it and the leadership and sense of liberty in the local community where one is able to live that way. Kudos to those who do it and the places it happens.

The Second Method

Understandably, some people are more comfortable with the second method.

It works too. A person stops wearing a mask and then asks permission to enter a place.

Some say it's a good way to honor the property owner by saying, "This is your store, may I enter?"

However, it is a bad way to honor yourself.

Man was not made to wear a polypropylene mask across his face.

Truth be told, if one operates a retail store, the presumption is that anyone off the street interested in spending money may enter, so this asking permission method really doesn't pay all that much honor to a property owner.

Additionally, there is, for whatever reason, an increased chance of this method failing.

Some people will tell you "No" to anything you ask them for. By default, they are predisposed to offer a negative response to virtually any question.

If Bob Barker[2] says "May I give you a car?" Those default-negative-response predisposed people might be expected to say, "No, I'm busy."

If Andrew Carnegie[3,4] says "May I give you a library?" Those people might be expected to say "No, leave me alone, weirdo."

If you ask, "May I enter without a face mask?" These people will predictably default to their standard answer: "No."

I fully encourage you to say to business owners, "I don't want to wear that stupid face mask because it doesn't work. So are you going to let me in to buy something or should I go to your competition during this recession and spend my hard-earned money helping them keep their doors open?"

I like this approach because, whatever you do, my suggestion is to not be a wuss about it.

You'd think reasonable evidence and peaceful cooperation would go a long way, but it doesn't. Not as far as I'd like at least.

It just doesn't work very well at this moment in time, which brings me to the third method.

I don't particularly like the third method. Yet the third method is the subject of the book.

Yes, that's right, I've written a book about a topic that I don't particularly care for, perhaps illustrating all the more importantly why the third method is so necessary.

The Third Method

The third method says a great deal about what a toxic society we live in.

Instead of peaceful cooperation, it calls on you to cite the law. It calls on you to try to pull rank. That is far from ideal.

Instead of the science behind the ineffectiveness of the masks, it calls on you to point to some piece of paper written by who knows who, signed by who knows who, with some official-looking seal on it, perhaps put there by who knows who, ostensibly read aloud at a press conference that you didn't attend, reported as the truth ad nauseum[5] by journalists and politicos you don't personally know and who have repeatedly proven themselves unreliable to those who pay the slightest bit of attention to the affairs of the world.

The third method lends credibility to all the wrong tendencies in our society.

But you know what, Rome wasn't built in a day,[6] and the awful direction of our society won't be course-corrected in a day.

I'm writing to get you through this day and to get you through it unmasked, with your proud face showing and your sense of individuality beaming through on full display, with your full respiratory system able to do the work it was created to do and to do that work unimpeded.

4

That's what I'm doing. I'm worrying about today, and I'm worrying about how much more wonderful our society will look once we worry day-by-day about getting through one more day with no face mask, linking day-after-day into a better way of life.

This is a hope that one-by-one, a person saying "How do I get through just one more day with no face mask?" will lead to noticeable change and course correction. We both know that a society can change drastically with just small beginnings. Person-by-person, giant change can take place.

It just needs to start with one individual holding a better standard for himself than what we've grown accustomed to.

The standard I recommend for this area of life is:

"Never again."

Vow today, to never again wear a face mask.

Never again.

If you make that your standard, if you make that a necessity in your life, the rest will fall into place and you will figure out what you need to do in order to never again find yourself in a face mask.

And I really mean never again.

The third option applies to many millions of people.

All it asks for you to do is something that many people aren't comfortable with, but which means a great deal: read the law.

Read the face mask laws.

Once you try to do that, you will probably be surprised to learn that there is no law.

Laws are passed by legislative bodies. Around face masks there are "orders," "policies," "statements," "guidances," "letters," "protocols," and many other official sounding words that do not mean the same as "laws."

This is a pretty good reason why hundreds of sheriffs[7,8] have publicly stated their refusal to enforce these glorified press releases.

Many more police departments and police officers quietly[9] refuse to enforce face mask policies.

If you are polite, you probably won't end up with a ticket or anything like that if you refuse to wear a mask when push comes to shove.

That means there may not be a legal consequence to plugging ahead with a store manager on face masks, even if they do get the police involved.

But that's a matter for another moment, and I very much caution against any unnecessary interaction with the police, because it can very unpredictably turn awful.

Though it is quite a significant distinction, let's temporarily overlook the fact that there are no laws on face masks.

Find The Source Document

The third method asks you, nonetheless, to find the source document and to give it a read, even if it is some silly policy made by some back room nobody. In doing so, you are re-enforcing the authority of that back room nobody, and I certainly have some reservations about that and where it leads, but again, I'm trying to get us through today. I won't make the good the enemy of the perfect, especially as I slog through the hell that 2020 has become and wonder what has happened to my country.

Where did everything go so wrong?

No, in the midst of that, in the midst of rallying the brave few, I won't worry about the back room tyrant having a newton more force behind his power, because I'm looking at the change that will be brought to lives, families, communities, and countries by a few more people a day going maskless and announcing themselves sovereign humans.

So, this third option is flawed, but it is also pretty good in a few ways.

One way is to enforce that we are people of the book, people of the law, literate people, people of records and history and knowledge that goes beyond the temporary storage of the brain and has a more lasting physical capacity on paper.

There is good reason memory has been called, the essence of civilization.

I want you to point to that paper — to say we have agreement and knowledge and methods that precede some guy at the door, or some store manager, or some gatekeeper, or some local public health official.

We have more than someone's temporary verbal slip of the tongue, when we demand in writing what a person is enforcing.

In writing we can look to it, and point to it, and cite it, and question it, and record it.

Written law is a powerful defense against tyranny. Written policy can be too.

It's not perfect. It can be a tool for tyranny as well, but it's pretty good.

Sometimes A Written Document Can Be A Lifeline

Science says there's no net benefit to wearing a face mask and it could be quite bad for both the mask wearer and those around him. Instead of altering their ways, in response to that science, hundreds of millions are at this moment masked.

We are at the edge of the abyss and we might have fallen off. I'm not sure.

If some back room bureaucrat's written policy is what I can use to get myself, and maybe you, back from the abyss, I will consider it a welcome life line.

This is a book about that life line.

I request you try your best to read this chapter and move on with life, resolving to never again wear a face mask.

The rest of the book, as mentioned in the introduction, is for those who aren't that swift, earnest, and ready for the immediate freedom that decision brings. They may need a little extra assurance.

The Steps In The Third Method

The third approach is as follows, quick and easy:

<u>Step 1</u>: Identify where you are going.

<u>Step 2</u>: Call them up.

<u>Step 3</u>: Enquire about the policy.

<u>Step 4</u>: Request an exemption under the policy.

<u>Step 5</u>: Confirm what time they can expect you.

<u>Step 6</u>: Have a look at their policy if you must.

<u>Step 7</u>: Request a more strongly worded exemption.

6 and 7 are nonsense that almost never have to occur.

1, 2, 3, 4, and 5 are simple and effective and are the ways I have gone shopping, gotten a haircut, entered a hospital, gone to doctor's appointment, and so much more with no mask.

That's not because I'm in South Dakota where there might not be face mask laws, but where plenty of people voluntarily mask themselves.

Nope. I'm in a very different environment.

I live and work in one of the very worst and most compliant face mask and lockdown locations on this planet. With myself as proof and thousands of happy people who have followed this method, let me elaborate 1 through 5 and let me leave 6 and 7 for a future chapter so the bold pursuers of freedom who need freedom right now like they need air in their lungs, can get on with their day unmasked, the first step forward of their life unmasked.

The One Sentence

Many millions of people are exempt from face masks.

If you are one of the millions with a medical exemption, be sure to mention one single sentence:

"I am unable to wear a face mask safely."

As an example of how leniently received these exemptions are, Sonoma[10] County California offers you an exemption if you have breathing difficulties. The state of Michigan, by order,[11] offers you an exemption on the honor system.

Thousands of policies have a similar level of leniency. Almost every policy that exists, offers lots of leniency and flexibility in its written version. Such policies merely require you invoke your exemption.

Apply that one sentence — *"I am unable to wear a face mask safely"* — with a few quick caveats and you are done wearing that mask.

That has been my experience. That has been the experience of thousands of others.

Now, I'm going to elaborate on a few of those caveats.

The Golden Rule

Everyone you encounter must be treated according to The Golden Rule:[12] do unto others as you would have them do unto you. Take it a step further, do unto others as you would have done to them.

Never raise your voice, never get into a shouting match, never show up at a face mask compliance checkpoint unprepared. The people checking don't deserve that stress and neither do you.

Come Prepared

Come prepared. That means you've spent ten minutes doing your homework before arriving at any checkpoint: you've called ahead, you've checked with a supervisor about exemptions to the face mask policy, you've determined that you fit the exemptions, you've asked for the exemption, and have received the exemption.

Name Drop

Name drop. Know who you are asking for at the door if something goes wrong.

Keep It Drama–Free

If there's drama you're doing it wrong. This is a low drama, low tension situation. You should never be caught on camera applying a face mask exemption because there should be nothing particularly noteworthy taking place.

Honor Your Privacy

You must treat your privacy as paramount. Don't answer questions about your claimed exemption. *"I am unable to wear a face mask safely,"* says everything you need to say.

Don't Avoid Life

If you are staying home in fear, avoiding essential activities out of discomfort, you must stop and apply your valid exemption. The world will be a better place if you do.

That's it.

If that makes sense, please close the book, commit to never again wearing a face mask, and go on your way.

If that does not yet seem crystal clear, the rest of the book is for you.

Method 1 And Method 2: Go At It With Bluster

Tensions are high. There are places that rather low-level employees have been told they are the "front line" in a war. This front line talk is destabilizing to many personalities, as it leads to an artificial inflation of their role in society.

An additional moral component has been added to this. Anyone who won't cooperate is evil. The unjustified claim that it is a moral issue to wear a face mask certainly escalates tension.

Making bluster further challenging, anyone monitoring compliance has gotten huge pushback from the public in massive shows of bluster. That's a lot of live action training. You will probably lose if you go head-to-head with a grocery store employee expecting him to read and interpret a legal matter while the face masked public and face masked staff are watching.

Those are key problems with Method One and Method Two. They may be ideal, but are not a good fit for the reality of many situations. Method Three is a relatively good fit for the reality of almost all situations.

Method Three: Bring This Up
In A Way That Cooler Minds Can Prevail

I'd recommend the phone, and I'd recommend calm tones, if your goal is to be able to shop maskless in order to avoid the breathing difficulties that wearing a mask might create for you.

You could say something like the following to a grocery store manager if it applied to you:

> "The San Francisco face mask order says that all people must wear a face mask in your business. That poses a problem for me, because I would not be able to wear a face mask, because I have a condition making it difficult to breathe while wearing a mask. Luckily, the order has an exemption for people just like me who cannot wear a face mask, because of a medical condition. So I'm calling to ask if I could come by today or tomorrow sometime and to have you guys follow the city order by having me not have to wear a face mask because of my condition?"

Pause for a bit. Give the manager time to think. Wait for him to let you know where he is with his thoughts. It's possible he has yet to hear that this is actually written into the order. Many people who are unable to wear face masks have probably already been turned away at the door of his business.

He may have some objections. If the following is true, it may also be helpful to offer. I know it is true for some people I have encountered.

> "…I can tell you about my condition if you'd like, if that is something you would need, but it would be my preference not to share that…"

"...I tried to get into my doctor for a note, to address my flare up and make this easier, but it was impossible. They aren't even answering their phones..."

He may say "No," but that happens very infrequently. Even in the most over-the-top compliant environments, a "No" from a manager is uncommon. Reasonable conversations about face masks lead to reasonable people saying "Yes," and may also lead to unreasonable people saying "Yes."

Managers Infrequently Say "No"

If he says "No," don't raise your voice. Don't threaten in any way. He's under a lot of pressure in his role. We all are. Don't speak about reporting anyone. Don't talk about lawsuits or government. This is a marathon, not a sprint. Take it easy. Pace yourself.

Recognize that it may be over his pay grade. Recognize that you don't want to get anyone in trouble and that he could get in trouble for letting you in the store. Just ask for a number to a supervisor. Perhaps even suggest that you call the supervisor together if that may help to disarm the situation.

If the supervisor says "No," do the same with their supervisor. Take down names and numbers and document the conversation. Go all the way to the CEO if needed. If the answer remains no, ask the CEO if you may speak with him and their general counsel.

From there you could go to your state's Attorney General. I know of at least one case working its way through the courts as we speak, in which a state Attorney General is standing up for the maskless. Going to an Attorney General is not my preferred option, but it is an option.

When one feels stuck in a situation, it can be quite empowering to recognize how many options actually exist.

Alternatively, you could just go to the competition, who may be more reasonable with your request for accommodation and more interested in your business.

The Difficulty Of Breathing
In A Face Mask Is Well-Established

I know it's frustrating to have to jump through these hoops just to go grocery shopping without wearing a mask that makes it difficult to breathe, dangerously difficult for some.

In 2018, Yolo County,[13] California posted cautionary advice about face masks before the wearing of face masks became so politicized in spring 2020:

> "N95 respirators can make it more difficult for the wearer to breathe due to carbon dioxide build up, which reduces the intake of oxygen, increased breathing rates and heart rates...N95 use may lead to increased heart rate, respiratory rate, work of breathing, carbon dioxide buildup

in micro-ambient air and heat stress — potentially posing risk to sensitive populations."[14,15]

A 2010 study[16] of ten healthcare workers in *Respiratory Care*, a monthly peer-reviewed medical journal, placed study participants on a treadmill for an hour showing that even with an exhalation vent, the carbon dioxide levels in an N-95 mask become far higher than would be allowed in a safe workplace and the oxygen levels far lower.[17]

On April 23, 2020, a driver in Lincoln Park, New Jersey lost consciousness, careened off the road, and crashed into a pole. Police found no signs of drug or alcohol use and believe that the accident was caused by driving in an N-95 face mask for several hours.[18-27]

Face masks aren't a cure-all and come with some meaningful downsides, especially for at-risk populations.

In fact, it's worth noting that face masks don't filter out small particles. A 2016 study of dental[28] uses of face masks points this out. Face masks can be useful for preventing direct, immediate contamination of a surface from a person who is coughing and sneezing, but the fine-particle aerosolized portion of matter is still transmitted.[29]

There's Little Benefit To Wearing A Face Mask To Protect From Covid

With so little benefit, it's actually pretty crazy to wear a face mask. And it's definitely crazy to elevate it to a moral standard as some people are doing. The puritanical American roots have turned on those who dare step outside with a full, unexposed face, just as they turned on the "witches" at Salem,[30] in a period of mass hysteria that will be forever remembered as a dark point in the American experiment.

Philosophical Reasons To Not Wear A Face Mask

There's great symbolism to saying you will or will not wear the face mask. Some go so far as to call them fear masks. Many appropriately descriptive names exist.

There is also another practical factor involved: it may be a burden for you and you may be legitimately exempt from wearing it while society figures out if the executive branch of government should have the authority to make these sweeping orders. You are, after all, the only person whose actions you are able to control.

If a face mask presents a health burden to you, look at the written policy of your face mask order, identify health or other exemptions, and establish clear boundaries around your wearing of that face mask.

You will be better off for having defended your own boundaries and your own wellbeing. And though this additional benefit may not be in your own self-interest, you will have helped others who have a similar hesitation around masks defend their health and safety, by merely defending your own boundaries on this matter.

Not only can courage be contagious. It can be benevolent as well.

The Lesson Applied

General Principles

Many millions cannot safely wear a face mask. With the one-size-fits-all face mask approaches, this presents a problem.

Those who cannot safely wear a face mask are pressured into wearing one, to their own detriment, or they are alternately, discouraged from using vital services due to the heavy-handed enforcement measures that place personal safety secondary at best.

The reasons for not being able to safely wear a face mask are many: from obvious issues such as chronic lung ailments and terminal heart conditions, to less obvious issues like panic attacks, dyspnea (shortness of breath), angina (chest pains), cephalalgia (headaches), migraines, internal physical deformations from injuries, or genetic abnormalities.

So Many Doctors Choose To Be Deaf To Their Patients On This Topic

The list of conditions that are suddenly becoming problematic due to face masks are so numerous that without specialty training, you would never even imagine them existing. Not even some doctors are hearing about them.

Hearing the arrogance of some doctors on this topic, dedicated to putting their egos first, their politics second, and their individual patient's wellbeing somewhere after that – it is no wonder so many people tell me they would never even bother trying to bring up the topic of face masks with their doctor.

People afflicted in this manner appear to be bearing the brunt of the problem quietly. Writers like me, who have taken a stand in favor of individuals and their individual medical concerns are hearing those stories though. The stories are at once heartbreaking and inspiring.

Heartbreaking, because of the sheer heartlessness being waged en masse as a society, as full compliance with face mask orders are being demanded at all cost. Inspiring, because so many people are standing up for themselves and their loved ones, despite the tremendous cost involved.

I hope to be able to tell more of those stories in future writings on the topic.

Best Practices Around Face Mask Exemptions Are Developing

In addition to my own experience, I have received many correspondences from people crossing face mask compliance checkpoints and sharing what works and doesn't work for them.

There are some behaviors that work repeatedly across-the-board, and there are some behaviors that don't work. Using these principles, I have yet to wear a face mask even one time.

Of course, on this constantly changing topic, it's important to keep nimble about what works and what doesn't work, rather than settling into too comfortable a behavior. This is especially necessary in our era in which so many turn to the twenty-four hour news cycle and social media for the "truth" of the hour.

There was a time when society could change minute-by-minute all it wanted, there were people wise and moral, well-grounded in what was true and in no need of a reporter to tell them.

Luckily, in this era there are such people like that who know the same truth today that they knew yesterday and didn't even need to turn on a television or pick up a newspaper to make sure that what they knew to be true yesterday is still true today.

Though we may feel like we live in a time of unprecedented flux, many of the same truths of reality are as true as they have ever been.

One truth is, no matter how bad things get, if you can find a way to relate to someone, one human to another, you may be more likely to get a human response.

One sentence is supremely helpful. You almost never need anything else, even in the most locked down environments: *"I am unable to wear a face mask safely."*

I'm going to elaborate more on why that is such an effective sentence, and often the only sentence you need at a compliance checkpoint.

The Risk Of Putting A Person In A Situation Where They Practically Have To Say "No," Is That They Say "No"

While those millions who cannot safely wear a face mask also have legitimate sovereignty concerns, constitutional concerns, natural rights concerns, legal concerns, and perhaps many other concerns, there are very few Americans policing face mask policy who will effectively quit their job for the benefit of another by saying

> "I totally agree with you, no one should have to wear a face mask, I'm going to look the other way knowing that I may be one of the unemployed 30% of Americans ten minutes from now by honoring your personal sovereignty."

That would be purely irresponsible of that person checking for compliance, and you would be expecting far too much of them. You'd probably be expecting more from them than you might expect from yourself, which isn't fair. That's hypocrisy, in fact.

You can, perhaps, imagine how ineffective it therefore is, to make such an argument at a compliance checkpoint. It's simply not the right venue.

The compliance checker may even have been trained to involve a supervisor anytime anyone makes such a natural rights claim and to have you added to a blacklist. To violate that instruction could again come at the cost of them losing their job. Great effort, after all, is made by management consultants and behavioral psychologists to create policies that remove the humanity from a human and to make him more like a machine while on the job.

Going the natural rights route is particularly dangerous because it is an axiomatic[31] battle. It requires the compliance checker to believe the same hard-won axioms as you. If they believe in anything, they are far more likely to accept the commonplace "For the greater good," combined with the anti-sciencey rhetoric of face mask enforcement and fear that floods the airwaves.

The places where you are most likely to find strict face mask enforcement are the places where you are least likely to happen upon someone who shares those axioms: coastal locations, big cities, airports, and a host of other hubs. You might end up with a memorable conversation, but in those places you aren't likely to get yourself through the door unmasked with that kind of approach.

While I have no cross-sectional data, I would also presume that those who self-select for jobs at compliance checkpoints are less likely to be sympathetic to natural rights.

The odds are against you with this argument in this venue.

Honor Your Own Privacy By Not Talking Specifics About Your Own Health & Wellbeing With Strangers

Other people who cannot safely wear a face mask, may have a face mask exemption for a medical reason that they are exceedingly comfortable talking with strangers about. A problem in that situation is that a stranger may not agree with you about the severity of your medical problem and its impact on you wearing a face mask. This is not a discussion to have with a stranger.

You open the door to questions like "Well, how bad is it really?" or statements like "It would mean a lot to the other customers if you would wear a face mask for the first ten minutes you are in the store, until you start to feel discomfort." Do not open a door to this line of conversation.

At a compliance checkpoint, some people who desire to pass by unmasked, will talk brashly about the *Americans with Disabilities Act* (ADA)[32] protecting them from having to disclose personal details. Others will talk about the *Health Insurance Portability and Accountability Act* (HIPAA).[33] I just choose to rely on standards of common decency and personal privacy. Although aspects of those laws are based on exactly that sense of decency, there is no need to invoke federal law. Medical advantages and disadvantages over others are a personal affair. Psychological advantages and disadvantages over others are a personal affair. Abilities and disabilities are a personal affair.

I recognize this sounds quaint in a time and place when people fly flags from their homes, tattoo their bodies, and wear handkerchiefs to publicly proclaim private matters such as their sexual proclivities or other momentary, aberrative behavior. However, the popularity of such displays does not change good sense and wise behavior around privacy. The wise man doesn't talk about his personal affairs with everyone he meets.

The personal is personal, and the public is public. No stranger is entitled an entry into your personal affairs. No matter how much this era wants to make everything public (except for the mischief of government, which we are assured in this era must always be as secret as possible for the wellbeing of all), it is the wise who maintain a solid division between personal and public.

The specifics of why you can't wear a face mask are nobody's business. Choosing to violate that basic concept of decency, puts you at a disadvantage at a compliance checkpoint.

Waving Laws Around Can Backfire Easily

Since pervasive laws can be detrimentally stumbled upon, a summary of applicable laws are part of the onboarding for any well-trained employee these days. It's useful to know applicable federal law in any field and how they are likely to impact an employee's training.

As one example, on the topic of face masks compliance, an employee isn't going to want to ask about your specific concerns that cause you to be exempt from wearing a face mask, because it opens them and their employer up to additional liability in the conversation.

Knowing that basic detail of training, makes it easier for you to simply say *"I am unable to wear a face mask safely,"* and to know that in many situations your privacy is going to be honored by the properly trained person checking for compliance. The path of least resistance is the path many employees will take.

The goal of this method is to allow any compliance checker a path of least resistance. When that path is properly offered, nearly all compliance checkers take it, and allow a person with a legitimate exemption to pass.

A goal of the method is to make your full noncompliance as easy on you and others as possible and to allow you to therefore never again wear a mask.

Some employees shutdown when they hear laws. Some employees call their supervisor. Some employees are trained to turn you away and report you directly to their legal department. Certainly, not all training is followed. Plenty of employees will totally disregard whatever was said at a mandatory training session at 8:30 a.m., four months ago, before they had their second cup of coffee that morning.

The more you press them with heady matters like laws or philosophy, the more your effort is likely to backfire.

Waving laws around can backfire, especially when it adds tension to a conversation.

That would be another way that people with legitimate exemptions put themselves at a disadvantage at a compliance checkpoint.

Escalation Can Backfire

Unless you've sized a person up and know what you're in for, don't try to go toe-to-toe with anyone manning a compliance checkpoint that you need to get to the other side of. The odds are against you. By autumn 2020 you won't have been the first to have gone toe-to-toe with them and lost.

If you don't need to get past them and just want to blow off some steam, that's an entirely different story. Go toe-to-toe. Have fun. That is not the situation I'm focusing on though.

This is a method for helping those who need to get past a checkpoint to do so successfully in almost all scenarios and to have their legitimate exemptions consistently recognized.

People enforcing face mask rules encounter resistance all day in adversarial settings and win. They have encountered that so much these past months, that some of them have become expert at it. Others don't like going toe-to-toe with a customer and consequently back down. There's little way to know who will be who.

Additionally, by this point in the process — more than 200 days after the first lockdowns began, and almost as long for mandatory masking orders — there are many redundancies built in at almost every checkpoint. You will eventually lose if you go toe-to-toe and escalate tension.

Insurance Companies Have Played A Role

Insurance companies have skilled actuaries that know how to use statistics in favor of the insurer. Insurance companies are consequently excellent at identifying cost-saving loopholes quickly after they appear.

Insured businesses have heard clearly that they will not be protected from Covid lawsuits by their insurers if they are lax in their enforcement of what is widely considered established science.

Perhaps after three years of costly legal battles with an insurance company, a business owner may be able to finally establish in a court of law that there is little science behind a face mask mandate. How many businesses owners and managers want to make that legal battle the next three years of their lives, especially against an insurance company with seemingly unlimited resources?

Such a sacrifice of three years of life would feel quixotic and with limited upside. Some are made for exactly that type of chore, but to expect it of everyone, or even many people, is out of touch with the realities of life.

Push the employee to do something that will invalidate insurance coverage, and you are putting yourself at a disadvantage at a compliance checkpoint.

If you can present your needs in a way that does not force them to violate their insurance policy, you allow the struggling business to survive another day, and to accommodate you.

Business Owners Have Bigger Battles To Fight, Like Staying Open

As private enterprise contracts, many business owners are concerning themselves with merely keeping the doors open. To do otherwise is to disregard their shareholders. Unless the shareholders themselves are pushing against face mask orders, it's unlikely the business will take a firm stand against mandatory face masks, whether it be mom and pop or a mega entity.

In that environment, it's quite hard to win toe-to-toe. Many people are just thinking about preserving their jobs and preserving their businesses, that even those who might have agreed in more prosperous times and who would have stuck their necks out, are unlikely to do so.

By all means, if you have outsized influence with such businesses, or special relationships that could sway the discussion, voice your concerns. These concerns are best voiced in calm settings, which is not likely to be at a checkpoint, but on the phone or by email ahead of time. Even more effectively these discussions can take place during a meal together, at a social event, or over a round of golf, all settings even further removed from the tension of the compliance checkpoint. In reduced tension settings, it is easier to hear and be heard. In those settings, life can feel less guarded, less zero sum, less black and white, and more cooperative.

What All People Manning
A Checkpoint Have In Common...

What they all have in common is their humanity. If you keep things nice and calm and you behave in a friendly way, virtually all people are going to respond favorably to you. If you keep the issue of your exemption nice and focused, by saying *"I am unable to wear a face mask safely,"* almost all people will make an exception for you. They won't ask questions. They won't give you a hard time. They won't ask much else.

There's a little bit of humanity left in many face mask policies. The humanity is in the exemptions around someone making the statement *"I am unable to wear a face mask safely."*

Someone working a checkpoint might say "So what?" or the equivalent, especially if you look healthy.

Stick with it and add a small clause, if you want: "I am exempt from your face mask policy, because *I am unable to wear a face mask safely*."

If they push further, you should feel comfortable saying "I am not comfortable talking about this private matter with others. *I am unable to wear a face mask safely.*"

If that doesn't work, simply say "May I speak to someone else?"

I strongly recommend no other conversation at a compliance checkpoint. Almost all other conversations are losing conversations. If you are yelling, you are probably doing it wrong. If a bystander is recording you in hopes that your outburst will go viral, you are probably doing it wrong.

Some compliance checkers might want to debate your condition. Some compliance checkers might want to see your doctor's note: the answer to that could be "Yes, of course I have a doctor's note." 75% of those who ask will stop there. They will not even ask to see the doctor's note. They only want to hear you say that you actually have one. If they press to see your doctor's note, you can say you don't want to show the note because it mentions a personal condition of yours that you wish not to share with strangers. That's common for many doctor's notes. Yours is not likely to be different from that. It makes the note more credible, but also unfortunately can be overly revealing about private matters.

If they really want to see your doctor's note, I recommend you just pull it up on your phone with the request

"Please don't read it too closely, it mentions a condition that I prefer to keep private."

No one wants to hold your dirty phone in their hands in the age of Covid. They will glance at your tiny screen, notice the legitimate-looking letterhead and the signature and will not even look further, themselves a little uncomfortable to have to go through the whole experience.

Seldom (perhaps 1 in 10,000) will the conversation go there if you treat the other person as kindly as possible and stick with *"I am unable to wear a face mask safely."*

Front Line

Many are so frightened of once commonplace activities such as touching another's phone to take a photo for a family or to shake a friend's hand. This fearful behavior is even more common among those referenced as front line[34] workers. The wide gap between the amount of bravery attributed to these front line workers and their irrational fear of a fairly common communicable disease is notable.

Never before have I known bravery to be synonymous with hypochondria.

Quite to the contrary, hypochondria was seen as a lamentable mental illness among people so out of touch with reality that few would take their concerns seriously.

An Additional Helpful Face Mask Exemption Phrase: "I Have A Medical Exemption From The County"

As local jurisdictions push face mask orders, and the media pushes guilt, and threats of fining businesses are bandied about, the decency behind *"I am unable to wear a face mask safely,"* has lost some of its appeal. Most importantly though, it was only ever designed to work in low conflict environments, or spoken over the telephone.

It comes with limitations. It may not be enough in a high conflict situation, which is one reason why I recommend against high conflict situations, but it's useful to have another phrase in your back pocket if needed: "I have a medical exemption from the county."

Every county order I have read has medical exemptions. The exemptions are massive. If you fit those exemptions, you clearly have a medical exemption from the county.

When you say that phrase, you are creating a shortcut that doesn't require anyone to think through why you say that you are exempt.

No, it simply tells the person what they need to know: "We don't need to worry about the county bogeyman."

They can breathe a sigh of relief upon hearing this statement from you.

The county bogeyman is who they fear. Every business owner does at this point. Some of the health departments in the 3,141[35] American counties have been real tyrants in the name of protecting people. The counties, by this point in Covid, have a lot of authority over considerable aspects of life in a way previously unknown to them.

Some officials return that power easily at the end of a crisis. Few do. Some citizens demand its return. Few do.

Your personal freedom from the action of any petty tyrant who may exist in your local county will still be a direct result of how effectively you are able to cause that freedom to rest in your hands.

By referencing the county you are speaking the language of the employee and their manager.

"I have a medical exemption" or "I have a medical exemption from the county" are clear, concise, effective statements for the tension of the checkpoint.

My preference far remains seeking low tension environments and defaulting to *"I am unable to wear a face mask safely."*

Why It Is Good To Let Cooler Minds Prevail

The Lesson seeks to have you negotiate this matter in a way that cooler minds can prevail. The more that can be done, the better off that likely is for the "little guy," in the exchange.

Anyone can ultimately refuse you service or entry.

The idea of letting cooler minds prevail keeps this in mind and seeks to extend the conversation as long as possible in your benefit and calmly, until you've found satisfactory resolution.

If someone manning a compliance checkpoint gets too worked up or gets too embarrassed in front of others or gets too proven wrong too brazenly, they might just shutdown.

Having that person shutdown is likely not in your best interest, especially if you have a dire need to cross his checkpoint.

Please Raise Cain, But Preferably Offsite

If you are treated unfairly, you can pretty easily make an employee's life a nightmare in this era. Make a few phone calls to supervisors. If that doesn't work, then work your way to the top of the company. This is so incredibly important. Call their superiors and then annoyingly follow up, preferably daily. That level of diligence is one way to get things done. Seldom is follow-up necessary. So often, a single three-minute phone call is enough.

Very few executives wake up in the morning and say "I hope to get bothered by a relentless, irate customer today." If you cross their path, they will almost certainly do their best to handle your matter so promptly and well that they will never again have reason to hear from you.

Only if you totally exhaust that process, only then consider going to the media, or using social media. Media and social media are not effective places to begin. Unwilling to do the effective work of picking up the phone, many people start with social media and end with social media. Used correctly, they can provide a lot of leverage, but often, social media and media are easy-to-ignore, ineffective, insulated ways to be easily muted.

Speaking To A Supervisor Is The Opposite Of Cancel Culture

Don't feel bad about going to a superior. This is the opposite of cancel culture. This is meritocracy. Cancel culture's adherents take your personal behavior, not committed in the commission of your job, and instead of walking away from you or engaging you on intellectual repartee, seek to report you to higher authority by getting you canceled from your job, canceled from your banking, or canceled from some other area of life, such as a communication platform. Cancel culture is an ethical and moral violation and harmful to free individuals in a free society.

In clear contrast, the world is benefitted when an employee who does wrong to you in the commission of his job is reported for doing wrong. It helps improve his training, or perhaps moves him out of that job and into another job to which he is better suited. It may help an entire company improve policy or may help to improve policy for the person who walks through that door to-morrow without a face mask.

"First world problems" is an unfortunate phrase used in the West to make fun of and mute valid criticism.

Complaining about first world problems is unlikely to benefit you as much as it is likely to shift policy to the benefit of others. It is a charitable and honorable thing to do, and many companies recognize that such feed-back is hard to solicit and valuable to receive.

The open and honest communication of personal dissat-isfaction can make life better for others. Dismissing that process, or first world problems, is just another example of nihilism. Honesty and feedback are concepts to em-brace, not ridicule.

You are right for reporting an employee who made your day a little worse with a face mask crackdown. Please do the world a favor and send that mini-tyrant home with an earful from his boss to mull over.

Figure Out What You Want Out Of This Exchange

The main problem that causes people to unsuccessfully cross face mask compliance checkpoints is that they have not decided on a clear outcome that they are working toward.

If you want to yell at someone at the top of your lungs in a public place about John Locke,[36] and to be the ridi-culed subject of a Young Turks[37] video that makes the rounds on Twitter,[38] with clips that perhaps the local Fox[39] affiliate also picks up, then these suggestions probably aren't for you. There's a lot of stress in the world right now. Vast portions of the globe are effectively living in a state of communism, without it being called such. I completely understand the need to blow off steam.

If you have a standard of wellbeing for yourself that specifically excludes the use of a face mask, and insists for yourself that you be allowed to go through your daily life without a face mask, then you are the audience for this method. *"I am unable to wear a face mask safely,"* is the easiest and most effective tool you can have at your disposal.

Many honorable people have made an unsuccessful ruckus at a checkpoint, but it seems that some of them really just wanted to go through the day without wearing a mask. That is sad. It doesn't have to be that way. This method is for them.

The act of making a ruckus and the act of successfully crossing a checkpoint unmasked are not always mutually exclusive, but are almost always mutually exclusive.

Seeing if you fit into one of the checkboxes, on a flowchart, that a corporate functionary needs to check off, will make it easier for you to pass. You make it easier for them to show you compassion. You may be one of the many millions who can simply say *"I am unable to wear a face mask safely,"* and will be left alone to cross the compliance checkpoint unmasked.

This lets you pass, and it lets them keep their job. It may not be perfect, but it provides for the primary want of each party to the interaction.

Insightful Economics Is Useful At A Moment Like This

Two people may appear to be in conflict, so what do they do? One answer is to seek to identify each other's primary wants and to seek to mutually provide for them as well as possible, even if that means eschewing the secondary wants that may be surrounded by higher levels of animation, but which are not at all primary, once a little conversation or other examination takes place. This mutual provisioning of primary wants is written of quite positively by Carl Menger in his 1871 classic *Principles of Economics* [40] which ushered in the field of modern economics.

Menger is the more impressive of the two Carl's to have been active in the field of economics in this period. The other being the far less impressive, but more popularly known Karl Marx.

Though Menger is not a household name, nor able to be universally quoted, even within the field of economics, Menger perfectly described so many aspects of peaceful human interaction in the many ways they lead to individual empowerment through cooperation of others.

The work of Karl Marx so effectively makes man a pawn at the hands of the powers that be, in any era of the last 170 years. The work of Carl Menger, so effectively makes man a king in his own kingdom, or a queen or a bishop or a pawn or whatever mutually agreed upon role is arrived upon.

To stop turning to Karl for economic suggestion and to start turning to Carl has untold impact on the individual who makes that transition, as he inevitably comes to free himself from the role of oppressed pawn.

Do You

People have pulled guns over face masks,[41] people have fought over face masks,[42-47] and I know of at least one shopper who has died over a face mask,[48-50] leaving a great absence in the world around the life of the deceased. It also leaves a great absence in the family and community of the father who pulled the trigger. Many lives will forever be altered for the worse by the horrible way that particular conflict at a face mask compliance checkpoint was resolved.

I imagine a world where this can be handled far differently. The maskholes demanding everyone mask up are insisting a personal medical issue be handled by fiat, which never goes well.

The level of force, intimidation, and ultimatum around this topic is very bad for society. Widespread inability to use words to settle a dispute is evidence of a devolution of culture. The face mask issue is the proving ground for greater areas of compliance to come. Unless good people cause the slippery slope to end here, masking up, deplatforming, and cancelling is not where this ends.

Less than 80 years ago, the United States government put Japanese Americans[51] convicted of no crime into prison en masse. Today, mainstream politicians and media in the United States are advocating for a political system that killed more than 100 million civilians[52-55] over the last century. Since *Roe v. Wade*, a number of babies equivalent to more than half of the current black population[56-59] have been aborted by the eugenicists who run and fund abortion clinics. A black baby in New York City[60] is more likely to be aborted than to make it out of the womb alive. The United States has almost constantly been at war[61] since its founding. All this barely begins to tell the story.

The United States government is awful. So many with their hands on the levers of power are awful. There is no moral backstop within the government. It doesn't come to an end with them. No one in DC is the deus ex machina.[62]

You are deceiving yourself if you don't think this can't get so much worse.

If you are one of the many millions affected by a mask, rather than wearing a harmful mask, now is the time to take a stand.

It doesn't stop everywhere until a mass of people insists it stops, but it can stop in your own life when you make it stop. You still have control over that in your own life.

I personally don't intend to make this my last stand, but for my own wellbeing I have not once complied with a face mask order, and I have no intention of ever complying with a face mask order.

How to Be Exempt From A Face Mask At The Grocery Store Every Time

Many write me about this topic. The most common face mask request I receive is how a person can exercise an exemption at their grocery store.

This has worked for me every time.

<u>Step 1</u>: Look up the store's phone number online.

<u>Step 2</u>: Take out a pad of paper, write the date, time, and phone number.

<u>Step 3</u>: Call and ask for the manager, writing down the name of anyone who says their own name to you, or any other name for that matter. "Oh, Melody will be back in about an hour," is a great excuse to copy down Melody's name. If asked, your reason for calling is that you have a question about the face mask policy. If the person on the phone claims sufficient authority over the topic, just talk to them.

<u>Step 4</u>: Say to them "*I am unable to wear a face mask safely*, … May I still shop with you? … I was thinking of coming by this afternoon."

<u>Step 5</u>: Be patient. Don't say anything. Let them have their turn. Don't interrupt. Listen. Take notes.

They will A: Say "Yes," B: Offer to shop for you, C: Say "No," D: Ask you more about your condition.

Step 6: If they say "Yes" (88% of the time), you are all done. Congratulations. That was easy. After completing the next step, just go shopping.

If they offer to shop for you (10% of time), get your shopping list and go to the store. Alternately, you can push back on them, explaining that you don't know what's offered at the store, so you obviously can't just make a shopping list. This will work better than half of the time.

If they ask about your condition, which they almost certainly won't (1% of time), tell them you aren't comfortable talking about it. There are lots of good reasons not to go down that road with them. If they say "No" (1% of time), ask to speak to someone else.

If you encounter one of the very few managers who deny you entry, and refuse to let you speak to someone else, please honor their property rights, go shop elsewhere, and try again during a different shift.

By all means, make it a point to also call their corporate office about the matter. There is only one regional grocery chain that I know of, in which the local manager would have the support of the corporate office on not being willing to entertain, let alone offer an exemption, and one national big box hardware store. Overwhelmingly, national offices recognize the valid need for exemptions.

Step 7: This is very important. Ask this: "So should I ask for someone at the door? Or what should I do when I arrive?" This is a question that will get you a higher level of service. The person on the phone will likely suggest you ask for them or another manager. Get the name of anyone you should ask for. Be sure to use that name when you arrive.

This is an important step, because often a manager doesn't want you standing in line unmasked; a manager doesn't want you freaking out other customers; a manager doesn't want you lingering around the store unhelped.

Because of this step, I am often escorted to the front of the line (some cities still have two hour long lines for groceries, and the people living there put up with it). Because of this step, my presence in the store will often be announced across the employee communication channels and employees will be instructed not to harass me, nor to allow anyone else to harass me. Because of this step, I am given white glove service at the grocery store, the same level of service I hope you are granted for your bravery. I've never in my life been treated like such a valuable customer at the grocery store as when I have invoked a face mask exemption.

Don't Cause A Scene

Please don't cause a scene. Calling ahead of time is the right way to do this. Tensions run high at the door. Approaching a face mask compliance checkpoint unmasked puts you at a disadvantage and may put the person manning the checkpoint unnecessarily on edge.

Don't Avoid The Trouble

Please don't avoid the trouble of making this phone call. This three-minute phone call is vital to the process. It peacefully, respectfully, and reasonably resists a one-size-fits-all medical order.

Don't Go Into The Store With A Mask

Please don't go into the store with a mask, even if you are just in a hurry. If you have a legitimate reason not to enter a store without a face mask, don't push yourself to wear it. Instead, push yourself to stand up for yourself and your legitimate and honorable boundaries. There is little that can be more important than spending five or ten extra minutes on this. Please vow today to never again wear a face mask at a store.

Some point out that freedom isn't free. No one is asking you to spend your Christmas in a fetid French trench. No one is asking you to storm Omaha Beach. No one is trying to get you to travel half a world away in the mind-numbing name of "defense," and to undergo all manner of horrors.

What I am asking, is that you take this unpopular stand and not wear a face mask if you are one of the many millions of exempt individuals.

Don't Avoid The Store

Don't avoid the grocery store. Don't avoid the unpleasantness of the phone call to a manager and the tiny risk of uncomfortable, but calm confrontation.

Your liberties are being incrementally denied you and denied many others. You are stopping the picking away at freedom with this seemingly tiny, but incredibly meaningful act.

How This Can End

When 100% of people stop complying with the face mask orders, the face mask orders are null. They'll be null long before then.

How This Can Get Worse

When 100% of people comply with face mask orders, there will be a goggles order, and a face shield order, and a visor order, and a hermetically sealed helmet order, and who knows what else.

You do the world a great favor when you don't wear a face mask. You do the world a favor when you fit into an exemption and live your life unmasked.

We already know the good science says that face masks do little against Covid.

We already know that improper use of a face mask may not just be a net neutral benefit, but may be a net negative.

In an era devoid of leadership, the people around you need someone to stand up and lead. Not by running for office, though that could work. Not by getting appointed to a government board, or sinecure, but that too could work. They need you to make it your priority to lead by example.

No other leadership is needed from you than this most vital and poignant leadership. In this era, be the finest version of you that you can be and if you excel, you will be your community's finest leader, for leadership does not come through appointment, but through acts admirable enough to want to be emulated by others.

In this specific situation, and in many others, you do so much good for the world by identifying your boundaries, communicating your boundaries, and defending your boundaries.

How To Invoke A Face Mask Exemption At The Doctor Or Dentist

Dear Mr. Stevo,

Thank you for the excellent article about not wearing the mask at the grocery store. Bravo! Neither have I, and each time we do so, we create just a little more precedent to exercise our God given Liberty.

I am scheduled to have a dental treatment shortly. Any advice you can offer about how not to comply with the mask mandate? It would be most appreciated. I don't intend to wear a mask under any circumstances, but neither do I wish to endanger my dentist's license to practice.

Blessings, and may Liberty increase forever!

– John S.

No one wants to cause their dentist to lose their license, and those with a legitimate face mask exemption don't want to put themselves at risk by wearing that mask. Your dentist's office has a face mask policy. As with any other face mask policy, you can learn about the policy and exemptions and see if it fits you.

In the same way that you need never wear a mask to the grocery store, there's no reason to wear a mask to the dentist or doctor when you have a legitimate exemption to their rule.

These are steps I would recommend for your dentist's office or doctor's office.

Step 1: Inquire About Exemptions

Over the phone or by email you can simply write "I am scheduled to come into your office and was wondering about the exemptions to your face mask policy."

Email and phone each have advantages. Phone allows for more flexible and direct interaction, easier reading of social cues, and greater ability to build rapport or exercise already built rapport.

If you are worried about not being ready to answer a question on the spot, then email may be the way to go since it will give you a little extra time to think over your response and to say what you need to.

Step 2: See If You Fit Their Policy

Take a look at the response. Honest human interaction is based on the idea of identifying your boundaries, communicating your boundaries, and defending your boundaries. You have now started a conversation in which you are able to communicate your boundaries and in which your dentist and his staff are able to communicate theirs. This is a good first step in the right direction.

Step 3: Request An Exemption

Ideally, they will send you a written policy, to which you can respond *"I am unable to wear a face mask safely."* A written policy sent to you is best because then you can clearly see where you fit into their policy and whether your exemption counts. It puts all patients on the same footing in terms of granting exemptions.

However, like any other small business, a dentist or doctor is likely to have more busy work than time to handle everything. It takes some doing to put together a written policy, so they might not have any policy to send you. They might write "Do you have a medical condition that stops you from wearing a face mask?"

You could respond to their email with *"I am unable to wear a face mask safely.* Can you make the proper arrangements for me to come in?"

They May Request Alternate PPE

In a medical or dental setting they are used to all kinds of personal protective equipment (PPE), so they might say that it's fine to not wear a face mask, but that you must wear some other type of PPE, such as a face shield.

With this introduction of a new form of PPE, you can now start the whole process over again. You may be one of the many millions who cannot safely wear a face shield either. In the example of a face shield, you can again respond "In your policy, what are your face shield exemptions?"

After they send you the exemptions, you can have a look to see if you fit the exemptions, and state "I am unable to wear a face shield safely. Can you make the proper arrangements for me to come in?"

Whatever type of exotic PPE that is suggested to you, I recommend the same process: "What are the exemptions in your policy around that?" followed by "I am unable to wear it safely," provided that applies to you. It applies to many millions.

Though it may be appealing to leap at the fact that a face shield worn on its own is not efficacious, and to ridicule the person and their suggestion, I encourage you to leave that topic alone.

The more a person suggests various alternate PPE for you to wear, rather than just dropping the whole subject and honoring your requested exemption, the more it becomes clear that it's about emotion, optics, and control rather than science, health, and safety.

Repeated suggestions like that speak volumes and call into question whether this is really someone who you want making decisions with you about your health.

Step 4: Confirm That When You Come In, The Exemption Will Be Honored

Congratulations. You are one step closer to being a little bit more generous with yourself by not forcing yourself into detrimental situations and by not avoiding essential activity.

Don't hurry off the phone yet.

Before you get off the phone, confirm how you should enter the office on the day of the appointment so that no one is surprised. You're going to want to get some instruction and a name to drop.

"On the day of the appointment, who will be there and what should I say to them about this conversation?"

Your correspondent will almost certainly say that they have already marked the file and have put a note next to your name in the appointment software and that you can just say you spoke to "Julie," or whatever the name of the person on the phone is.

The Divisive Media

A trillion dollar media machine has been steadily at work for months, attempting to get consumers of information to automatically associate the unmasked individual with mistrust and a host of other negative sentiments. If there is any conflict on the day of your appointment, being able to recall and speak Julie's name will go a long way in simplifying the encounter and building trust.

Privacy Concerns & Strangers

No stranger deserves the trust of hearing about your personal concerns, including the person you don't know guarding the door at the grocery store. He has absolutely no business hearing anything more than *"I am unable to wear a face mask safely."*

Even that is none of his business, but that's the world we temporarily live in, and I am writing about how to continue life with some normalcy in that world. There is no reason for the question "Why?" to be asked or answered.

It is a harder situation, though, when the person you've known for decades and who has been a trusted source for medical advice is involved. If you really trust your doctor, and believe he is entirely scientific in his thought process and immune from the emotion and politics that has come to pervade nearly everything today, he is the one person you should consider listening to about face masks. Few doctors like that exist.

"I Would Rather Speak To The Doctor About This"

If a member of the dentist's or doctor's staff pushes you about details of your requested exemption, you may say "It is private, if I need to discuss it over the phone, I'd rather speak to the doctor about this."

Though it's a sincere stance to take, that will probably be enough for the issue to be dropped, as everyone tends to be quite busy in a doctor's office.

Your Dentist Needs To Know Your Medical Concerns

Your dentist is going to have every right to know if you have a heart condition or lung condition that is going to need attention while you are in his chair. He can hardly do his job right without knowing that. You put yourself at risk hiding such details from a dentist.

Though there are many medical conditions that prevent a person from wearing a face mask, other non-medical conditions should be kept in mind as well, since so many people suffer from them, and they are so very debilitating.

The Crippling Effects Of Panic Attacks[63]

Those who suffer from anxiety, panic attacks, and claustrophobia are beginning to speak up about their needs to live unmasked. The National Institute of Mental Health estimates that 4.7% of US adults, or 15,510,000, will experience a panic disorder at some time in their lives. An estimated 2.7% of US adults experienced a panic disorder over the last year, or 8,910,000.

That's a lot of people for a one-size-fits-all face mask mandate. It doesn't begin to take into account the panic attacks suffered by those with social anxiety disorder, depression, post-traumatic stress disorder, and many other conditions.

Face masks won't trigger all of those people. In fact, one aspect of panic disorders is that the trigger is not often evident. Before everyone is forced into a face mask, a transparent and vigorous public discussion should be had about the grievous harm that causes. Mandatory masking harms many people in many ways. Medical decisions are necessarily individual. One-size-fits-all approaches does not serve a patient well.

While panic attacks are generally not believed to be physically harmful, they have physical manifestations and can be the scariest physical experience some have ever had. To those who experience them, they feel very real. As the psychosomatic nature of panic attacks begin to attract further attention and research, the physical harm of panic attacks is likely to become more clear.

Maintaining Some Privacy Around Panic Attacks

Dentists and doctors are used to prying into a patient's medical history in order to identify potential dangers. Your dentist or doctor may really push to know more about your history of panic attacks or other conditions. You can talk about it freely, if you believe that serves you well. Alternately, you can offer him a statement like this that doesn't even mention the word panic attacks:

> "It's not a medical issue. It's more of a psycho-logical thing that I am currently working through. If you'd be willing to let me leave it at

that, I would appreciate it, but the bottom line is, *I am unable to wear a face mask safely.*"

Or just say the single phrase "Panic attacks." If the dentist or doctor keeps asking questions, you can simply say "Don't want to talk about it."

A Quick Summary, To Protect Against Probing Questions That Might Catch You Off Guard

Any probing questions like: "Who are you seeing?" "Are you getting treatment?" "How long has this been going on for?" "Can I call your therapist and confer with him?" can just be answered with "I'd prefer not to talk about it right now."

Any PPE suggestions can be answered with "What is your exemption policy?" You shouldn't have too much more to worry about.

Say "No"

"Thanks for your email, would you please send me referrals to three other practices." That's the only sentence I would send to a dentist who told me "No."

Dentists are able to work with all kinds of communicable diseases and to use all forms of protocol to protect themselves from a sick or potentially infectious patient.

Hepatitis and HIV are two examples that have given dentists considerable worry in recent years. Covid is nowhere near as concerning from a biological perspective.

They should have no difficulty accommodating your desire to pass from the front door to the treatment room unmasked.

After you get your referrals, call those dentists and make sure you are clear that you are interviewing dentists, considering becoming a new patient, and will be unable to wear a mask. There are plenty of dentists who will be happy to earn your business by providing you with the experience that you want.

Please Don't Wear A Mask

Truthfully, many people look better in masks. They look more comfortable. Some even have a level of comfort that showing their face to the world and to their family doesn't provide for them. That's a truly sad thing to be able to say.

Considering that, you might understand the existential threat you pose to such people by suggesting anyone should be unmasked. If it becomes abnormal to wear a mask, they will need to go back to not wearing a mask. They wouldn't have the courage to do otherwise. By being an individual, you deny them that strength in numbers. Considering this, you might understand why they tell so many stories about society's duty to wear masks.

The reality is, too many Americans are harmed by the awful, one-size-fits-all mask approach and its heavy-handed enforcement.

The world is made a better place by making sure those who qualify for an exemption speak up and take that exemption. "...We create just a little more precedent to exercise our God given Liberty."

I have not worn a mask and don't intend to, recognizing the detriment it poses to me.

Face Masks In Public

In public, just as in private, you can figure out the exemption and figure how you fit into it. If you fit into it, go about your day complying with the law under your exemption. It's as simple as that.

No one with an exemption should be expected to do otherwise. A great deal of societal pressure is being levied toward a one-size-fits-all approach. You deserve the ability to craft your own approach as an individual, with individual concerns. Luckily, every order I have seen leaves plenty of room for individuals who will take the time to educate themselves about such orders and then identity any valid exemptions.

A great deal of compliance takes place simply because people with valid exemptions will not take the time to determine how they fit into those orders.

Consequently, I have heard from formerly active people who have become shut-ins and have, in other ways, isolated themselves from a healthy lifestyle, merely because they didn't realize that there might be an exemption in the lockdown and face mask orders and policies that apply to them.

It is not in society's interest to have such people live as shut-ins and certainly not in the interest of those individuals.

Luckily, we have not reached a state of tyranny where the orders make no such consideration for the wellbeing of individuals.

Allow your personal rights to invoke a legitimate exemption to lapse unused by you and we may see society fall into precisely that kind of tyranny.

Face Masks In Church

It's been said that singing spreads germs.

Some people use that as a reason to put an end to their singing.

It's notable that living also spreads germs.

Would the same people resolve to stop living in a desperate effort to reduce the spread of germs?

Others have suggested that to leave churches open, to go unmasked, to come within six feet of a fellow Christian is to put God to the test.

Some would say the Church should lead the way. Leadership is wonderful, but church "leadership" in the age of Covid has been some of the most cowardly, secular, bootlicking nonsense that has nothing to do with Christ, such as closing the sanctuary, the place where the faithful have long sought refuge from the tribulations of the world. This is a penny wise and pound foolish approach to Christianity, which is hypocritical at best, and seeks to intentionally subvert the Church to secular forces rather than act as servant to God. The two are exclusive. Only one master can be served.

One of the great joys of being a Christian is the amount of strength it gives you to stand in the lion's den, the amount of bravery it gives you to appear before Nebuchadnezzar, the amount of courage it gives you to be a stutterer speaking before the mighty pharaoh.

Do not negate those powerful rewards of faith by being cowardly. There is no justification for the master. Life brings with it risks. That's no reason to stop living life. It's all the more reason to live as well as you can, walking in God's steps and walking courageously.

It would be no surprise to the faithful to know that devout Jews and Muslims, too, feel that they can move mountains because of their faith.

Cowardice among the faithful is misplaced.

If you've honored the Sabbath every week for decades of your life by going to the seat of your congregation and worshipping, and the last ten generations of your family have done the same, is the best response really to stop that behavior?

The answer is no.

The Church is the last behavior you should stop. Let it only be stopped by your death at life's end.

Be a courageous member of your faith community, who is not easily frazzled. Let your faith be the rock solid foundation upon which your life is built, even if the rest of the world around you is choosing to build their lives on sand.

The place you should most insist upon not wearing a face mask is your church.

Face Masks At Protests

It is said that chanting and congregating can spread germs. Of course it can. There is no activity in life that will not spread germs.

Victorian Bifurcation Of Life

It is a strange Victorian sentiment in us that seeks to delineate the clean from the dirty. Life has gradients.

Not every organism is pathogenic to a human.

No pathogenic organism will do harm every time it comes in contact with a human. Life is a balance of risk and reward.

Even if we could eliminate biological risk by eliminating all exposure to micro-organisms, what trade-offs would need to take place in such an antiseptic world?

We know already what havoc antibiotics wreak in man when they are used to create an antiseptic internal environment.

We know, too, what havoc cleaning products wreak in man as they are used to create an antiseptic external environment.

The research is just beginning to scratch the surface in those areas, but it looks like the Victorian tendencies to draw a clear line between clean and dirty, with all micro-organisms placed solidly on the dirty side of that line is not only poorly informed, but also harmful.

The Micro-Organisms Are A Part Of Us

The micro-organisms are part of us. In our contemporary culture that has oversimplified the concept of majority rule, the notion that our bodies are a majority not human cells, but instead non-human micro-organisms should give pause to those who would draw such a line.

The micro-organisms, even the pathogenic ones, are a part of our microbiome. That microbiome is arguably a part of us. That microbiome is almost certainly part of what keeps us healthy.

This strange reductionist tendency in contemporary Western culture, to so stringently divide clean from dirty, in a way that is so clearly harmful to individual human life, must be avoided.

As we begin to understand that there are little creatures, so numerous, living in and around us, and as our technology becomes more attuned to identifying them, we must not have a knee-jerk reaction at the sudden awakening to the previously unknown.

The Primitive Nature Of Knee-Jerk Reactions

This is the most stultifying, primitive approach that a people claiming to be educated can have: jumping to fear as the primary reaction.

The knee-jerk jump to fear says little about the data and a great deal about the person choosing to take that jump to fear.

Please do everyone a favor and calm down before you attempt to assess the data. If you can't calm down, please do everyone a favor and excuse yourself from having a vociferous opinion on this matter.

Just because there is a technology said to be able to sense the presence of Covid-19, just because we have rapid testing, just because we can identify some symptoms, does not make it okay to suddenly blow all manner of life out of proportion because our leadership — governmental and civil — lack the ability to perceive the world in proportion.

It is not a lack of scientific knowledge that so disables us in 2020. It is not a lack of data. it is not a lack of study or research.

It is a lack of philosophy. It is a lack of thoughtfulness. It is a lack of reason that so disables us.

We have easy access to the data. We have little wisdom among our leadership with which to process it.

This weird reaction should be no surprise when a society places the asocial nerds of the culture in charge. These are technocrats, brainiacs, and really quite flamboyant folks who would not survive in a more meritocratic environment.

How Badly Can The Technocrats Screw This Up?

How badly can they screw things up? 2020 is living proof. And boy do they hope you don't catch on to what's happening and run them out of town.

Do they want all manner of effective protest to come to an end because of Covid? Of course they do. They never wanted to hear your opinions to begin with. The technocrats have such contempt for you and your opinion.

They know who should run the world, and it's not you.

They are the only ones who should be able to chant and congregate. Only they should be able to approve what messaging is chanted and congregated around. You are not permitted to do so.

They have always believed that and now have a gimmick by which to manipulate you into believing the same and acting accordingly. Whether you believe it or not, the end effect is the same if you follow their edicts: the silencing of you and anyone else who doesn't precisely parrot the prescribed groupthink of the technocrat.

Precisely Parroting The Prescribed Group-Think

I do really mean that the parroting must be precise if you intend to go that route. Just look at Robert F. Kennedy Jr., a lifelong Democratic Party loyalist, and almost down-the-line adherent to stated Democratic Party values and technocratic ideals, with one exception — he thinks vaccines should be safety tested. Because of that single divergence from the party line, he is treated as a pariah.

RFK Jr. is the finest example of the level of compliance demanded by the American technocratic class. He is a Kennedy and a son of an assassinated attorney general and presidential hopeful, a scion of American royalty. It's hard to be any more party line than him and his entire story, but because of his one divergence he is treated entirely divergent.

The Choice Is Yours

It is your choice whether or not you comply. If you were already a person of spirit and character, how sad for you, and those around you, even the world, if you do comply.

If you were already a well-programmed and obedient drone, then there is little loss to you, me, or anyone else if you comply.

The choice is yours.

I know how I have chosen and will continue to choose.

I know directly how hundreds and thousands have chosen and by extrapolation how millions and globally billions of others have chosen.

And that's why I don't care, for my own wellbeing, how you personally choose, because I know there are enough others to replace you if you chose poorly and make yourself into a drone.

For you though, for your own wellbeing, if you want my opinion, which is what you likely want if you picked up this book – you must kick and scream and fight with everything you've got to not become the drone that modernity and its technocrats want you to be.

You must instead, at every turn, chose to be the life-affirming you that you can be.

Face Masks While Exercising

To the best of my recollection, every face mask order I've read offers an exemption for someone exercising.

There are many human activities that can be considered exercise and virtually all human activities benefit from additional fresh air.

Like all other parts of the book, if you like to exercise without a mask 1.) identify the order, 2.) identify where you fit into that order, and then 3.) invoke your exemption. That should be the work done in almost all situations.

A reader writes:

> "You are an interesting guy. 'Liberated' if you will. The thing that I love most is that you were maskless in a town that mandates masks. The people in San Luis Obispo wear masks in their cars while driving alone."

The question would follow, should anyone wear a mask when they are outside going for a walk to strengthen the body and get fresh air?

The people who do, appear to not be aware of the importance of fresh air and sunshine for human health. They additionally do not appear to be aware of the research apparent since January 2020 that points to Covid-19 as an illness contracted and spread in the home setting far more than in the community setting, such as schools, grocery stores, or outside.

Face mask policies and lockdown policies consequently do not rest on the science. Because of how Covid-19 is spread the science demonstrates a lockdown, the forced increase of multigenerational groups in a family setting, to be the exact wrong approach.

One should not be surprised when a far off bureaucrat who does not know you, has not examined you, and cannot possibly care a lick about you in all but the most theoretical of senses, cannot even care about your wellness. In that scenario, the bureaucrat of course creates a one-size-fits-all policy that causes you harm when enforced.

That awful system is what we have made into the norm across society and that many intend to increasingly make the norm. It does not take a rocket scientist to see what an obvious failure this method promises to be. In fact, the more educated a person is, the more likely they seem to be to fall for such awful "solutions."

The technocratic class has often failed society with their solutions. From the sociopathic "solutions" offered by World War II era governments in which individuals were not treated as inviolable, to the eerily similar "solutions" for Covid-19, in which individuals are not treated as inviolable. We can be sure that technocrat's solutions will fail when they do not treat individuals as inviolable.

History is littered with stories of how such anti-human, anti-individual technocrats will fail big whenever they are given the slightest bit of power.

It is up to you, the individual to watch, out for yourself and your loved ones, irrespective of the suggestions of bureaucrats.

You must not let someone with no "skin in the game" in your personal life, make dictations of your personal life, especially in such drastic scenarios as this.

Bureaucrats must be relegated to decision-making that matters to no one, such as whether the bureaucrat will wear blue socks that day or black socks.

Matters of your own wellbeing must be sorted out for yourself and by those trusted people you turn to for advice. That is part of the cost and joy of living in a free society.

The bureaucrat who you do not know cannot, by definition, be a trusted person. It is therefore entirely irresponsible to consider their advice as trusted.

Face Masks
In Government Buildings

A nice thing about government is that very few people in government positions care about much. That general disinterest may be an inadvertent source of greater human freedom. That being said, in government, there tends to be a protocol for everything. You are likely to be able to identify the protocol and are also likely to be able to use the protocol to your advantage once you know it. "You really aren't supposed to ask me about my disability, but I'll tell you if you really want," is probably enough to remind government functionaries to watch their boundaries.

In a different setting it would be different. Most people in government get that there's no point in caring. They are there to punch the clock until it's time to collect a pension. The quicker they realize that, the better it is for them. Often that is the direction that the available incentives push them in, and that their more veteran colleagues encourage them towards.

Face Masks And Jury Duty

Like any government entity, courts are likely to have clear rules and policies.

Courts have the ability to make accommodation for this scenario, but those that work the jury selection process tend to have a series of boxes to sort a person into, which makes this easier and are likely to quickly exclude you and return you to the jury pool in the future.

I've heard one account of not being able to wear a face mask being enough to keep a person from not going into the courtroom for jury duty.

If you strongly desire jury duty, you can first identify who at the courthouse can help you seek exemption or accommodation. Then once obtained, notify the jury pool supervisor that you've sought accommodation, had your accommodation accepted, and will be coming in unmasked for jury duty in line with the accommodation and to fulfill your civic duty to help others receive a fair and impartial trial before a jury of their peers.

Face Masks
On Public Transportation

This can be a tough one, because you are in a confined space.

To rob, beat, burgle, or shoot heroin in front of children on the playground and on the street, are not crimes that get enforced in San Francisco, but to go unmasked on public transportation can be a very different matter.

Such hypocrisy.

In the face of that hypocrisy, I recommend against simply pushing yourself through the door and instead taking the recommended approach in this book.

Each police officer has significant discretion in the exercise of his duties.

The standard for arrest is likely much lower when you are using a government facility, such as public transportation.

On the other hand, there is a long-standing history of accommodation for people with disabilities being made on public transportation. The same is true in these times related to Covid-19 exemptions on some public transportation systems.

The lesson applies to riding public transportation with a mask, just as it applies to all other areas of life.

Governmental programs can be so filled with the careful following of laws and policies that you may even have an easier time obtaining a face mask exemption in a government-run transportation system.

A significant caveat exists though: you are putting yourself in a government-controlled box — a subway car, a bus, a light rail car — and provoking the attention of men with badges and guns who have the right and responsibility to place you in a government-controlled cage — a jail.

That's not the front on which I seek to spend my life fighting this fight. The odds are stacked too far against the free man in that scenario.

Kudos to those who navigate that scenario and do it successfully, and I know of dozens who have.

It's merely a situation that demands a lot more finesse and a lot less bluster, because bluster can backfire so easily in that situation.

Interactions with police can be prone to unpredictable outcomes.

How To Invoke A Face Mask Exemption At The Barber & Get VIP Treatment

Dear Mr. Stevo,

Thanks for all of your writing on how to use a medical exemption to end these face mask orders.

I walked by the barber the other day, and he's got a sign up saying you need to wear a face mask.

I can't safely wear a face mask, but I don't know how to say that.

– Gaynelle F., Vallejo, California

Short answer: Just tell him.

Long answer:

Do you have any idea how many fine pieces of hair a barber inhales each day? This is not to mention the hair product, chemical treatments, skin cells and anything else that's in your hair, made airborne by him preening you.

It can be a dusty business.

Plenty of barbers have these little nagging tickles in the throat and lightly cough in response to that irritation. The light cough would have gone unnoticed before the age of Covid. Who knows what kind of reaction it might garner today.

Your barber may have always wanted to wear a mask. He just never wanted to freak you out, so he didn't.

More barbers are going to start wearing them, not entirely because of Covid either, they can now avoid breathing some of that stuff, without freaking out customers. In fact, in this era, he might even look virtuous doing so.

Barbers Are Economic Barometers & Calipers Of Public Sentiment

Barbers tend to be quite entrepreneurial. That is the nature of their business.

Barbers know rent intimately. They know taxes intimately. They know regulation intimately. They know their daily, weekly, and monthly nut. And they know customers intimately. They are in touch with what is happening in an economy and community and tend to be realistic and personable people.

Barbers have not seen a normal customer-load for more than half-a-year, and that has been a big setback for them.

Barbers, after all, are people with financial plans.

It's no surprise that barbers were the ones leading the charge against the lockdowns in Michigan, Pennsylvania, Texas and other places.

They are at once service providers and valuable glue to a community, deeply in touch with their customers' needs and wants. At least that describes any barber I've ever known. Not only that, but in the barber chair you are vulnerable, you can share sensitive details about your appearance there, and you can get your barber's advice about it. There can be an intimacy and trust to that relationship that doesn't exist in most other business relationships.

If You Can't Be Direct With Your Barber, Who Can You Be Direct With?

If you can tell your barber honestly and openly about a strange hair that keeps popping up in the weirdest place, that you've never told anyone else about, it shouldn't be too hard to speak to your barber and tell him you will be unable to wear a mask.

He wants your business, and he will make an exception. If he is worried that your exemption will be bad for business and scare off other customers, he'll probably happily open up for you an hour early by appointment or stay an hour after close for you.

It's A Great Time To Be Generous With Yourself And Others

If he does that, give the guy a few extra bucks, or even better, bring him a gift he's sure to love. It could be a bottle of the kind you might give him at Christmastime, or some cigars — something he can take home, and show to the wife, while bragging to the rest of the family about what great customers he has.

You do that, and you'll buy ages of goodwill with the man. And heck, a gift like that is deserved if your barber is anything like the amazing barbers who I've trusted enough to sit in their barber chairs all these years. It's not just about the goodwill. It's about doing a solid for someone who has probably done you so many over the years, and in the present time, the more emotional generosity and financial generosity we can offer those around us, the more we are helping to ease some of the stresses that so many are presently going through.

The world could use more generosity right now and less divisiveness. You may not be able to change the world, but this very moment you can decide to bring a lot more emotional kindness to your corner of the world.

Exempting Yourself From Face Mask Rules At The Barber Shop

Just like any other business with a face mask order, you just need to identify your boundaries, communicate your boundaries, and defend your boundaries by 1.) identifying the face mask rule in question, 2.) inquiring about exemptions, 3.) seeing if you fit into those exemptions, and 4.) communicating and confirming your legitimate exemption. That can be changed a little with the informal and friendly Joe, who runs his own shop and has no flowchart that he must follow.

Usually, the statement "*I'm unable to wear a face mask safely,*" is a useful tool to invoke a legitimate exemption to a face mask rule. With your barber, who is practically the opposite of a faceless corporate drone obediently following a flowchart, it makes sense to be more human in your approach.

Step 1: Bring Up The Topic

"Joe, this is Stevo. I was walking by and noticed you got this face mask sign posted up."

Let Joe talk.

Step 2: Inquire About Exemptions

"Joe you got any exemptions to this face mask rule? Cuz I really want a haircut, and I can't wear a face mask. The doctor says it's bad for my health. The doctor says 'Stevo, do not wear a face mask!' I'm just listening to the doctor."

Let Joe talk.

This second step might end here, or you might need to continue the discussion a little more. Alternately, you can offer to call back a little later after he's had time to think about it. Calling back later would be my approach. It's a more understanding way to deal with the various pressures of the situation Joe finds himself in.

Unlike the corporate drone, Joe has had better things to do than get training on face mask compliance. It makes sense he would need time to think, and he might be having a busy day with a long line of customers.

Whatever you do, don't get testy with Joe. A lot of folks have had success steamrolling face mask compliance checkers at checkpoints. Though it's not the method that I think works best, it might make sense for some people in some situations. I'd never do that with my relationship with Joe. He's a good guy and a reasonable guy. There's no need for anything remotely resembling steamrolling.

Step 3: Confirm With Your Barber The Procedure You've Just Heard Him Say

"Okay, Joe, so if I show up at 7 p.m. on Tuesday, you can make room for me, and I won't have to wear a face mask. Do you want me to give you a call that morning and remind you?"

Barbershops Are Tribal Gathering Places

Do all this over the phone and it will be a lot less tense. Barber shops can be like man caves. Once the rhythm of the tribe sets in at a barbershop, the easy background music gets to playing, and the people get to talking, a pecking order gets established, a mood, a rapport. Wherever you have a few customers or a few chairs, it seems to happen.

Whenever a new person walks in, the newcomer disrupts that vibe. That happens on a normal day in any tight-knit barbershop in a close community.

Imagine how much worse it is to walk into a barbershop where ten guys, dutifully wearing their masks, are shooting the bull about these guys who "won't wear a face mask, because they are too darn selfish," or some other media talking point.

If you enter into that environment and you put Joe on the spot in front of all those others, you're stacking the deck against yourself.

Joe loves his customers, but Joe hasn't kept his place open 27 years and put three daughters through college by getting into petty little disputes with everyone watching.

Do Joe a favor and let him talk this through with you over the phone, on his own terms, and with as much discretion as he chooses to use.

Draw A Line Today…

If you've got a legitimate exemption, do yourself a favor and vow to never wear a mask again. At some point you've got to draw a line: you can't go through the misery of the mask or the isolation of avoiding going outside forever. Why not cross that line now?

Start with your next barber appointment. If Joe can't extend you that customer service favor of not requiring that you be masked, there are other barbers who will.

Heck, half the barbers and stylists are running around making house calls these days, they've been given such a rough go by government. Joe is probably so interested in your business, he might even do house calls for you if asked.

These mask orders are bad news. More superstition than science, they are the wrong way for policy to be crafted. That's not me claiming that, that's 2016 research, now scrubbed from the internet, that describes how ineffective face masks are.

It was an enlightening piece entitled "Why Face Masks Don't Work," filled with lots of common sense, long known to the dental community, about the limits of face masks and a welcome piece of data-driven writing that came from a time before our heavily politicized era, causing it to quickly appear far more reliable than anything widely circulated since the politicization of face masks.

That journal article has been replaced by its original publisher with this Orwellian creepiness:[64]

> "If you are looking for 'Why Face Masks Don't Work: A Revealing Review' by John Hardie, BDS, MSc, PhD, FRCDC, it has been removed. The content was published in 2016 and is no longer relevant in our current climate."[65]

Thank goodness for the Wayback Machine,[66] which allows the internet to have an archived "memory," rather than to have inconvenient articles from the past descend down the "memory hole" made famous in George Orwell's cautionary tale about the future, *1984*.

The deeper into 2020 we get, the more it seems that the technocratic class has missed the intent of the book and turns to *1984* as an instruction manual.

...Or It Won't Stop Here

Something tells me the weird, Covid directives from government won't end there either. We're already seeing the evidence that places that were locked down fared worse, the same, or better than places that weren't. It seems more and more evident that lockdowns weren't the variable.

The Lesson Is Intended
To Be Applied In Every Situation

Human action is fluid and unpredictable. It's a beautiful part of life. I can't predict the future nor can anyone else. What we are all called on to do is this:

Identify our boundaries. Communicate our boundaries. Defend our boundaries.

In the area of face masks, if you have an exemption that means you are always doing the following:

Step 1: Politely inquiring about the exemptions to the policy.

Step 2: Politely requesting to patronize the business under the exemption.

Step 3: Clarifying that you will not be wearing a face mask and when you can be expected to arrive.

Step 4: Confirming what you should do when you arrive.

Step 5: Following through and maintaining a very kind, but firm exterior that will be incredibly accommodating, within your boundaries, while maintaining a firm certainty at your boundaries.

The intent of The Lesson is that it can be applied across all situations. It is a realization that honesty requires you to communicate your boundaries to another and to then speak them to another in a way that allows you to be heard by the other party.

Alternatively, you may just walk away from the other party.

Making this decision is vital for being an honest person. Decision at its root means "to cut off from."

One who decides, cuts off all possibility to later return to the previous way. There is a clear cutting off of one in favor of another.

This moment of decision is poorly honored in our culture at present. What is more desirable culturewide is to keep all options open. What is even more popularly desirable is to keep all options open at all times.

What is far more common than being decisive is to tolerate a person, to not communicate boundaries, to allow boundaries to be traversed, and finally in frustration having some type of meltdown.

This is the way of American society in this period in history, a way exported widely to all individuals of the world with a desire to be westernized.

It is a supremely dishonest way of dealing with others. Our overly literal era is obsessed with the telling of the details of the truth. Well, that's really very hard, and human communication is not black and white. There clearly are lies but not all that exist in the grey is a lie. Our overly literal era obsesses on the letter of the truth while being in near complete disregard for the spirit of the truth.

Are you honest about drawing boundaries? Will you speak hard details to the people who you find the greatest discomfort in speaking them with?

There is such great contradiction in American society in which grand life changing aspects of life are ignored, while the most minor and insufficient details are obsessed over.

This is a supreme example of living for the letter of the law and not the spirit of the law. Some people major in the most minor details and then walk away very pleased with themselves, though they have in the process involved themselves in the greatest lies.

The Lesson exists to forsake minor lies as merely irrelevant and to focus on the major lies. Neither lie is good, but when one has a log in one's own eye, it is no time to focus on the speck in your neighbor's eye, nor is it any time to focus on the speck in one's own eye.

Identify the log. Focus on the log. That is The Lesson. That is how a thinking person behaves who seeks to live a moral life.

To be mired in pedantry and legalism is to allow oneself to miss the grand moments of life.

Identify your boundaries, communicate your boundaries, and defend your boundaries.

You cannot be a fully functioning member of any community without doing precisely that. To do otherwise is to live a grand lie, no matter how much pedantic detail you follow in the face of people pleasing authority, demanding such disabling pedantry from you.

Focus on your own boundaries and you identify yourself and free yourself. This is a most vital tool on the teetering edge of the abyss we currently inhabit.

"Mandatory" Doesn't Really Mean Mandatory

English has turned to mush at the hands of mushy-brained bureaucrats and technocrats and consequently, those who are not mushy-brained are put at a significant disadvantage in conversation when they interpret the words of the mushy-brained as the words of the able-minded.

Words in English have so lost their meaning. This can be seen all around. One example is among young people — not yet having been entirely acculturated to the absolute lies of the empire that is American civilization and its outposts around the world. They find themselves in disbelief at how little the English language is useful at communicating the simplest ideas honestly and clearly.

Consequently, because of this devaluation of the effectiveness of words, there is an "inflation" that takes place among young people who are just trying to highlight important topics by saying the equivalent of "Hey, pay attention to this!"

What was once able to be stated as "Mercury is toxic," now needs to be stated more often as "Mercury is really very toxic," or increasingly "Mercury can literally kill you, like literally."

The word toxic has lost some meaning. The imperatives of the language have lost meaning. The verbal exclamation points of the language have lost meaning. The word "literally" gets overused as well, at times even being misapplied. In its use, you can make fun of a young person, or you can see a fellow slave on this awful anti-thought plantation on which we exist, holding up the once honed and sharp English language and wondering why the darn dull thing can't be very easily used to communicate.

Hardly can a young person be blamed for attempting to navigate a case of linguistic and cognitive degradation that they have only recently entered into.

Ernest Hemingway tried to strip the language of artifice and to use it to communicate clearly. He won a Nobel Prize in literature for this, but he failed to use language to think clearly. His life was punctuated with romance for the evil of socialism. Had he surrounded himself with a better crowd and better ideas, with his finely honed writing, how he could have soared as a timeless literary intellectual, but his philosophical foundation was so erroneous.

George Carlin called on people to end this linguistic inflationary madness in their own lives, saying that too many words were being used to communicate, simple, clear ideas and that the use of too many words to express a concept was not expressive at all, but undermines communication and is just another example of hiding the truth.

"People use extra words to make things sound more important than they really are," said Carlin in one appearance.

In another talk about the misery caused by using euphemism to dull the language, Carlin said[67]

> "I bet you, if we'd have still been calling it shell shock, some of them Viet Nam veterans might have gotten the attention they needed at the time. But it didn't happen, and one of the reasons is because we were using that soft language, that language that takes the life out of life. And it is a function of time, it does keep getting worse."

Word inflation is all around us in the English language and words have lost so much of their meaning. I have a suggestion on how to navigate some of this.

Examples Of Word Inflation And Effective Ways To React

As a diligent student of the contemporary face mask orders, it is my strong recommendation that every reader of a compliance order view the word "mandatory" when spoken by a bureaucrat or functionary as "recommended."

The phrase **"Absolutely no exceptions!"** means "Mask are advised, talk with us if that's a problem."

"You will be fined if you don't comply!!!" means "We'd really like you to wear your mask, but we probably have no legal authority, nor the will to fine you, especially if you claim any of the eight different exemptions to this policy, but we'd just like to express to you, and mainly to our insurance company, how incredibly serious we are about this policy, like literally."

The sentence "You will literally kill people if you don't wear a mask!" is similarly a demonstration of this word inflation, but it is also a cautionary message that is different from the others. It should be read as "We believe the crazy fake news, and we are unhinged. The media is more trusted than science. Perception is more important than fact. As such, we are more dangerous and destructive to society than Covid itself." It's my recommendation that you not interact with anyone posting such a sign, until they've had a long, sober vacation from the media cycle and an opportunity to calm down after the 2020 elections. Timeless wisdom is applicable here: "Beware. You never know what could happen when you walk through the front door of a person, who is like, really, pretty, basically crazy."

"Absolutely no exceptions!" means "We have a lot of exemptions."

"Absolutely no exceptions!" alongside threatening, flashy, original graphics means "We have a lot of exemptions, and we also have too big of a workforce with too much time on their hands at all levels of the company, not just the forty-nine-person graphic design team that made this sign, and consequently, you can expect both our third and fourth quarter earnings reports to be woefully out of touch with the earnings estimates of the street. Buy puts on our stock now."

"You must wear a mask in this store!" means "If you walk in this store twenty times without a mask, you might get called out about it three times, and we aren't even sure if our employees will even have the courage, interest, or stamina to do that even three out of twenty times, so we posted this strongly worded sign in hopes that it would deter you, even though we know that it probably won't deter you at all, but it may deter some people, according to a focus group conducted by a marketing consulting firm that our industry trade group's Director of Communications hired to give her twenty-six-year-old, out-of-work niece something to do during the economic downturn caused by the entirely overblown governmental corona response, so our General Counsel's assistant decided to post this sign at the front door of every single one of our chains based on a Friday afternoon statement from our momentarily distracted General Counsel in passing, in which she said with a very distracted and disinterested shrug three minutes before going out of town for a long weekend 'I don't know, I guess it can't hurt.' This was interpreted by her assistant as 'Immediately print this and post it at all entrances of all 1,048 locations nationally. ASAP. PDQ. Like, now!'"

Yes. These signs mean all kinds of things, but in the context of a time and place where "literally" doesn't actually mean "literally," the signs shouldn't be taken so seriously and should never ever, under any circumstance, be read literally.

Don't Take Face Mask Orders Too Seriously

All that is to say, "Don't take face mask 'orders' too seriously." Face mask orders are guidelines at best. In almost every situation, with all but the most rabid ideologues, you will get your exemption honored.

The problem with a rabid ideologue is that they believe their own hokum. Anyone who believes the hokum and falls for the narrative is doing themselves a serious disfavor.

A small selection of face mask crisis pragmatists. Just look to the pragmatic out there if you want to see how not serious these face mask orders are.

You see, some savvy people are using Covid to take an extended vacation for themselves. They are happily letting the world fall for it all. Don't expect them to protest.

Other savvy people are using it for their political gain, like Joe Biden or Kamala Harris who have called for people to just wear their masks until Biden beats Trump.[68] Don't expect them to protest face mask orders. Domestic disquiet is believed by pundits to helps voters usher in change. Some politicians wake up tickled upon hearing the news that yet another city burned overnight.

The vaccine manufacturers love the lockdowns because they can assure high vaccine compliance and low herd immunity rates by the time a vaccine becomes available. Don't expect them to protest face mask rules.

I've identified about two dozen other groups in society who like face masks: ranging from 1.) **the media**,[69] who desperately seek sensationalism to boost viewership numbers, to 2.) **the dishonest**,[70] who feel more comfortable lying with a covered face to 3.) **the ugly**,[71] who, let's face it, look a lot better in a veiled face, to 4.) **the dramatic**,[72] who, like something to get worked up about.

You can't expect members of any of these special interest groups to offer opposition to face mask orders. There are so many others too. They are riding the wave and will be ready to ride the next wave. No fuss. They see right through the hokum, but are happy to let things continue as is.

How To Invoke A Face Mask Exemption At The Veterinarian

Dear Mr. Stevo,

Just wanted to thank you again for your advice and encouragement regarding resistance to mandatory mask mandates.

I have an appointment with my vet this week. The vet clinic has a "mandatory" mask requirement, with which I do not intend to comply.

So I emailed the clinic an inquiry this weekend, and not having gotten a reply yet, I called and stated my concerns about not being able to wear a mask safely, as you suggested in several of your articles. The person to whom I spoke was most friendly and solicitous.

Turns out the "mandatory" mask policy refers to the parking lot, since the clinic is not allowing pet owners inside, mask or not.

Or in other words, the mask policy is essentially meaningless. Strike a blow for freedom, because every act of resistance makes it a little easier to assert our rights both for ourselves and for others who wish to live as free people.

Thanks again. Liberty!

– John S.

Just like any other situation in which someone is claiming authority over you, a face mask requirement at the veterinarian's office can be handled like this.

<u>Step 1</u>: **Familiarize yourself with the face mask order.** This can be done as simply as stating one sentence to an office manager or receptionist over the phone — "I see you have a face mask requirement" — followed by a period of listening to their response.

<u>Step 2</u>: **Educate yourself about the exemptions.** This can be done with a quick sentence — "Do you have any exemptions to this requirement?" — followed by quietly listening to the response.

<u>Step 3</u>: **If required, cite your reason for needing an exemption.** A good, clear, concise sentence to use is *"I am unable to wear a face mask safely."* This can be followed by a period of listening. There's really no need to get more in depth than that.

<u>Step 4</u>: **Confirm the details of the conversation.** You can make sure you understood everything clearly and that everyone is in agreement on how to proceed, with a statement like this "Okay, so I can just come to your front door at 2 p.m. today and mention your name at the door, along with this conversation, and there should be no problem, is that right?"

The Maskholes Who Want A Fully Masked Society Do Not Hold The Moral High Ground

This same process can be done for goggle requirements, face shield requirements, temperature testing, and all manner of other invasions for which you may have a valid exemption. Many millions are exempt, but rather than invoking their exemptions are struggling through the suffering of the dehumanizing process. As they quietly struggle they are told, "You are evil if you even think about not wearing a mask." Really?

A one-size-fits-all, heavy-handed medical approach for all people regardless of impact is the real evil. And I beg you to fight it, do it for yourself, because if you don't take a stand, it won't end here.

Caution: Unopposed orders by out-of-touch bureaucrats lead to more unopposed orders by out-of-touch bureaucrats.

The Governor of Maine, Janet Mills,[73] on August 14, 2020, ordered the wearing of what are effectively dog cones by restaurant servers as part of her "COVID19 Prevention Checklist Industry Guidance." The person who has successfully fought the face mask and learned how to say "No," will likewise be ready to take on this Twilight-Zone-like[74] challenge. Those who don't, are assured to see how very twisted the minds of their unchecked elected officials are. Until there is resistance, the policies and enforcement promise to get weirder and weirder.

If you have a valid exemption, I encourage you to follow this simple process at the veterinarian or anywhere else to boldly put an end to this tyranny in your own life.

You deserve better than to allow yourself to be cowed into harming yourself. You'd never allow such low standards of self-care for a loved one. Why would you allow those low standards for yourself?

The San Francisco Policy Analyzed

Face masks are being turned to as a largely superstitious solution to the concerns about coronavirus, as opposed to a solution driven by data. The data also indicates that the use of face masks comes with drawbacks.

That being the case, local orders requiring a face mask are likely to make clear that there are exemptions to the order.

The San Francisco Department of Public Health has played a leading role in Northern California, nationally, and globally in shaping corona response policy.[75,76] That official order along with directives from City Hall deserve further attention, as it makes notable exemptions to who must wear the mask.

It Is Dangerous For Children
Under 2 To Wear A Face Mask

Sudden Infant Death Syndrome (SIDS)[77] is a poorly explained phenomenon that frightens parents. Corona prevention or not, any artificial obstruction of a child's breathing goes against years of warning on this topic and flies in the face of the fact that some children do appear to inexplicably and permanently stop breathing.

The San Francisco face mask directives wisely state "Children under 2 years old must not wear a face covering. They may suffocate."

Children Under 12 Must Be Supervised,
And The Order Will Not Be Enforced For Them

The same caution around little ones up to the age of 12 is expressed in the San Francisco directives.

> "Children 3 to 12 years old are not required to wear a face covering. If they do, they should be supervised by an adult. Supervision may look different based on the age and maturity of the child. For some children, having a discussion may be enough. For younger children, parents and caretakers should be present during use by the child. Parents and caregivers should use their judgement."

The mayor of San Francisco has advised that this order will not be enforced for children up to and including the age of 12.

If You Have Documentation From
A Doctor Then You Don't Have To Wear One

Understandably, enforcement of the order is made easier if those with an exemption can show medical documentation. The San Francisco face mask order states: "If you have documentation showing a medical professional has told you not to wear a face covering, you do not have to wear one."

But that poses a problem because many doctor's offices have been shuttered. It is very difficult to get in to visit with a doctor. Therefore, the order also includes those who do not have a note from a doctor.

Even With No Documentation, If You Have Trouble Breathing, You Don't Have To Wear A Face Mask

Since not everyone can go to a doctor, you are exempt from having a doctor's note if a face mask gives you trouble breathing. According to the San Francisco order:

"Anyone who has trouble breathing, or is not able to take off a face covering without help, should not wear one."

Physical Disabilities Exempt You From Wearing A Face Mask

According to the City of San Francisco, "If you have a physical disability that prevents you from wearing a face covering, you do not have to wear one."

The ADA Protects You From Having To Disclose Your Disabilities

Please forgive the murky waters I'm about to enter as I attempt to identity leverage you may have in defending your boundaries in this matter.

The *Americans with Disabilities Act,*[78] drafted under Ronald Reagan,[79] passed through a Democratic Congress,[80] and signed by George H.W. Bush[81] in 1990, has turned into a massive governmental over-reach and assault on property rights. There are far better ways to address the needs of disabled individuals.

That does not change the fact that it is the law of the land, and whether or not it is law, remains at the core of many corporate training manuals: a properly trained manager doesn't want to give the slightest indication that he is being nosy about your health or disabilities.

Many people who suffer from disabilities find it difficult to talk about their disabilities to every person from whom they request accommodation. When you cite a disability, people may look at you in disbelief and request that you prove your disability.

In many situations, as the ADA has been interpreted, you are not required to disclose your medical condition to anyone. The Department of Justice ADA information and reporting line is 1-800-514-0301. Specialists are available at that number to apply ADA concerns to specific situations.

This poorly constructed law can be kept in mind for a point of reference related to how corporations train staff.

There's really no need to even mention this law. It's just good to know that simply saying "I do not want to discuss these personal details," or "I do not want to talk about the particulars of my health," or "I do not want to discuss my disabilities with you," almost anyone will back down and redirect the conversation elsewhere, either out of a sense of decency or out of desire to comply with a law that they may now realize they have skirted.

The Law Is On Your Side, Now What Do You Do?

If you put your local face mask order and the ADA together and are nice about it, ideally over the phone, it will probably work.

All you really need to do though, in almost all situations, is to say, *"I'm unable to wear a face mask safely,"* and ask for accommodation.

How To Fly The Friendly Skies With Your Friendly, Maskless Face

The airlines have quickly become a choke point for the face mask orders.

On the ground you have a choice. If Walgreens[82] turns you away, you can go to CVS.[83] If CVS turns you away, you can go to the locally owned place. If Menards[84] turns you away, you can go to Lowe's.[85] If Lowe's turns you away, you can order online. If Sprouts[86] turns you away, you can go to a farmers market.[87] If the farmers market turns you away, you can go meet the farmer around back and buy what you need out of the back of his truck. Most of those places don't turn people away, anyway, at least not if you invoke an exemption.

As predicted, the lockdown doesn't end when some blue ribbon panel says it ends. The lockdown comes to an end as every locked down person individually determines that they will return to living life normally again. Each day becomes more and more normal.

In The Air, It's A Little Different

In the air, it's a little different. It's not different because a passenger is captive. It's different because there is effectively no competition.

When there's virtually no competition in an industry, that often points to one of two scenarios:

Step 1: A product is the best that anyone could come up with and the cheapest and it makes everyone so incredibly happy that no one would ever even dare challenge the single provider of that amazing good or service. That does not describe the commercial aviation industry in the United States.

The other option is that:

Step 2: Government thugs and government mandates weigh so heavily on an industry that there is little competition in that industry, and barriers to entry are nearly impossible to surmount, so the consumer is left without a business that can provide the consumer exactly what he or she wants. Unfortunately for consumers, that describes commercial aviation, banking, healthcare, and many other industries.

Entrepreneurs want to work long hours to please customers in all manner of ways, unfortunately in those listed industries, sick people and government stand in the way of that help, as anti-consumer activists, anti-joy authoritarians, anti-satisfaction puritans, anti-fun police, and impoverishment enablers intervene in an industry to the great detriment of consumers.

Don't Get Caught Speaking Tropes Like "Monopoly" Or "Free Rider Problem"

But there is one industry that it doesn't even come close to describing: the internet. Many people call Google and Facebook "monopolies." Please don't be one of those people.

Monopolies exist when a company makes everyone as happy as possible, or when a government protects a big player from competition. Neither takes place in tech, at least not yet.

There's lots of competition for Google and Facebook. Some of the competition is pretty awful, and the consumer correspondingly chooses to use Google and Facebook, which makes those two incredibly powerful, but it is not a marketplace deserving of being called a monopoly.

When you call things a monopoly, or when you argue that externalities are bad, or when you call "free riders," a "problem," as in the common business school phrase "the free rider problem," you work against freedom.

Don't fall for it.

When you make that mistake, you invite a bigger government to step into your world in a more magnified way, and boy will they figure out a way to screw up whatever they touch.

If you want to know why all the airlines are behaving lockstep in line with each other, a meaningful reason is because there's nearly no competition in the airline industry, which is because of government's protective involvement in the industry.

Tyrannical Government Behaves Tyrannically

As can be expected, the face mask choke point is taking place in this heavily regulated anti-competitive industry.

Government and the corresponding lack of competition is one of the causes of this.

There's a positive aspect here too. As we've already covered, you know that there's always an exemption. Let's go through that a little.

The Same Four Steps Will Help You Through This Problem

True to The Lesson, that means you are doing this or some variation of this:

Step 1: Check the written face mask exemption policy.

Step 2: Figure out how you fit into the face mask exemptions.

Step 3: Requests your exemption.

Step 4: Confirm the details of how you fit.

Obfuscation Of Information Makes These Four Steps Really Hard, But Why?

At this point, I am more knowledgeable about airline face mask orders than any of the dozens of airline employees I've ever spoken to about the topic. Most employees trust Fox, CNN, NPR, or whatever garbage news source they pretend to learn about reality from.

That means, even those tasked with checking people in at the airport will say things like "There are absolutely no exemptions!" even though their airline actually has exemptions and it's their job to inform customers of them and facilitate those exemptions.

The lady at the counter will have a very different understanding of the rule than the guy you spoke to on the phone at 5 p.m. on Tuesday, who will, in turn, have a very different understanding of the rule than the guy you spoke to on the phone at 5:17 p.m. on Tuesday, even though they all may have gone through the same training.

"Why is this?" you may ask.

For some two decades, United has made it impossible for anyone to walk through an airport without humming the 1924 classic "Rhapsody in Blue"[88] by composer George Gershwin. The marketing departments of the airlines know how to communicate a message. If a message is poorly communicated by an airline, it's either because no one in the corporate hierarchy cares enough to communicate it well, or because someone decided that it should be poorly communicated.

Airline employees intimately connected to this topic have informed me that the latter is true.

"But, why is this?" Well, for goodness sake, the answer is because no one has a clue what they are doing, and they are pretty sure that their policies won't stand up to legal scrutiny.

In the true standard of corporate avoidance, the lack of leadership on this important topic is in full recognition that the longer they can avoid being the one chosen as the test case by the courts, the better it is for all potentially culpable people at an airline.

The insurance company has one view. The legal team has three views that are in clear dispute with each other. The C-Suite thinks something else. And none of them wants to make a gutsy decision, just like almost everyone else in this awful, cowardly land since on or about the Ides of March 2020 when the United States descended into a state of corona communism.

The big airlines are very difficult to get a straight answer from. Luckily, I've spent enough time traveling during this lockdown to still have gotten through my life without wearing a face mask, despite living in the most locked down city on this planet.

I've got a two-point plan for those who are entirely unable to fly with a face mask on.

<u>Step 1</u>: If you've got a medical exemption, use it.

<u>Step 2</u>: Beef jerky and chewing gum.

These are two methods that have shown a great deal of success for plenty of people.

If You Need A Medical Exemption, Just Use Delta & Bring A Doctor's Note

Most large airlines in the United States not only tell you that they don't offer medical exemptions, they actually follow through with it.

Luckily, one airline still has a somewhat clear face mask exemption policy. Delta. The following is, more-or-less, what you can expect.

If you walk up to the ticket counter and claim a medical exemption, about 1-in-5 employees will be trained well enough on the topic to not yell at you "No exemption!" while trying to hand you a clean face mask with their grimy hands from their big, uncovered, not sterile stack of surgical masks and waving it in your face.

If you don't talk to the correct employee among the five, you just need to keep persisting politely, until someone finally says to the correct person "This guy wants a face mask exemption. We don't have face mask exemptions do we?" Eventually someone behind the counter will step forward and say, "I'll handle it."

What will happen next, is that you will be asked if you have an exemption. Then you will be put on a telephone to speak to a Delta doctor at the University of Pittsburgh. The Delta doctor will ask you some questions such as:

"What is your age?"

"Why do you think you are unable to fly with a face mask?"

"Do you have a doctor's note?"

"Are you currently being treated for this condition?"

"What medicines are you taking?"

"What techniques have you used to try to tolerate a face mask?"

"How long can you tolerate wearing a mask for?"

Feel free to answer or decline to answer any of them. Also, at any time you feel uncomfortable in this process, you are likely to be able to decline to board and get a full refund from Delta on your ticket.

If you have a doctor's note that says something like this, you might get an exemption from the Delta doctor.

> "This man has severe advanced heart disease. We have exhausted all options for alleviating his difficulty breathing. He must not be asked to wear a mask at all. He is safe to fly."

Or if you have a note that says the following, then that request from your doctor might be honored.

> "This woman has severe advanced lung disease. We have exhausted all options for alleviating her difficulty breathing. She must not be asked to wear a mask for more than 5 out of every 20 minutes. She is safe to fly."

What If You Don't Have A Doctor's Note?

Even if you don't have a doctor's note like that, you might still be able to fly without a mask.

If you suffer panic attacks while wearing a mask and you speak about your difficulty breathing to the Delta doctor on the phone, and you don't have a doctor's note, and you've had this problem for years, and it's always been under control, and you don't take medicine for it, and haven't needed to see the doctor for it for many years, and the face masks have been a real problem for you, then you might be offered an opportunity to board the flight and remove your mask every five minutes out of 30 minutes or every five minutes out of 60 minutes.

You won't be able to go maskless. You'll need to agree to alternate between the mask on and off.

This "doctor" on the phone with you isn't so much a doctor as he is Delta's face mask compliance and negotiation specialist. His job on the phone seems to be to convince you to only take off your face mask every 25 minutes. He is a gatekeeper. Tell him that 5 minutes out of every 10 minutes would be better. Settle for whatever his counter offer is, thank him for his time, and then pass the phone back to the ticket agent.

You're supposed to allot an additional one hour for this process, but it really takes around seven minutes.

That leg of the solution is then handled.

It's very unlikely anyone will time you along the way.

If there is anyone along the way who you will see for less than five minutes, this will get you past them. If they give you a hard time, which they probably won't, just say 'Delta says it's okay,' or 'I have an accommodation.' That will probably be enough.

Now this does not handle the whole problem. This may only get you through TSA, into the lounge, through the gate, and onto the plane unmasked.

The next step of the plan may be required in order to go fully unmasked the entire time.

Some have been able to travel undisturbed and unmasked without the next step, but the next step is a handy insurance policy for those with a legitimate exemption, who cannot wear a face mask safely.

Beef Jerky And Chewing Gum

Have you ever chewed a piece of gum for an hour? I have. I've also watched others do the same. It's hard to tell what the person is actually chewing when they are chewing gum.

Have you ever chewed beef jerky? I have. That stuff can be a real jaw workout. I've also watched others do the same. It's hard to tell what a person is chewing when they are chewing beef jerky.

Airline face mask orders have exemptions for eating and drinking. You can't drink water every ten seconds for a three-hour flight, because you'll either run out of water or explode. But you can do something that creates the same visual effect: this fine fellow is busy eating or drinking.

You can open a bag of beef jerky on your lap, put a stick of gum in your mouth, and every time you are asked to remask can point to the beef jerky or your moving jaw. If you want to take it even further you can say "I'm eating."

The Thing You Can't Say

If anyone says to you "Are you refusing to wear a mask?" say "I was cleared by a Delta doctor," or "I'm eating."

Do not say "Yes, I refuse to wear a mask." If you refuse to wear a mask, you probably won't be able to board your return flight. Delta claims to have blacklisted 150 flyers as of late August 2020 for refusing to wear a mask.

I have no idea when the Covid fear campaign and face masks will end, though Misters Biden and Trump seem to both believe that face masks will be done by mid-November 2020. It would be awful if it went on longer and you ended up banned long-term from one of the airlines in this already anti-competitive industry, simply because you misspoke.

Call First

Before traveling, do your best to make sure that the telehealth "Clearance-to-Fly" system is still in place at

Delta. That's what this process is called. It won't last forever. Something else will replace it.

The big airlines, true to their heavily regulated methods of protecting themselves from consumer-pleasing competition, have been clamoring for a face mask mandate from the federal government, which the White House, to date, has refused to grant.

Delta's Best Phone Number For Face Masks

I have found this phone number to be Delta's most useful customer service contact on this topic:[89]

"Customers worldwide with general questions or concerns regarding services for those traveling with a disability can contact Delta at 404-209-3434."

They won't be able to answer many details, but they should be able to tell you with some accuracy if the face mask exemptions and the Delta "Clearance-to-Fly" program are still in effect, since they are more likely to interact with the program than the average customer service representative at Delta. All US airlines likely have a similar team.

The same page on delta.com cites "14 CFR Part 382,"[90] a federal law entitled "Non-Discrimination on the Basis of Disability in Air Travel," a topic that some people have chosen to delve deeper on: face masks exemptions and discrimination on the bases of disability in air travel, as an alternate path. I have not. Beef jerky and chewing gum are effective enough.

The Hoops One Must Jump Through
To Have Their Legitimate Exemptions Honored

The airlines are unfortunately very close to an across-the-board ban on face mask exemptions. There's not a lot of wiggle room. Millions of people have a legitimate face mask exemption for legitimate conditions. Yet the government-protected airline industry is nearly lockstep saying to those millions of people "Stay home!"

That's awful.

If you can't wear a face mask, they want you to stay home. If you still persist, they want you to be entirely unaware of the process, so unaware that you don't even want to take the risk of traveling. If that doesn't get you, they put out press releases saying that you could be one of those 150 banned passengers if you try to fly without a mask. If you indefatigably persist after that total obfuscation, they will use a phone call with a Delta-paid doctor, who has no allegiance to you, to use the authority of his white coat to bully you into doing something that could be dangerous for you.

That's just another step toward the idea that we are not individuals, that medical interventions should be determined by plebiscite, that your neighbor should have just as much of a say about your own body as you do.

Fluoride in the water, mosquito abatement, other mass spraying of chemicals, statins in the water, forced vaccines, face masks for all, and so many other topics —

these are personal medical decisions that some believe should be levied across entire populations by vote, at the behest of the public health profession.

They are the same band of anti-social and destructive technocrats, Marxists, communitarians, and others who plunged us into the ongoing six months of economic and human misery claiming that they needed to implement corona communism to save 2 million Americans in 2020, an entirely false and disproven claim. The further away from the Ides of March 2020, and more sober we get, the more evident it becomes that the people entrusted to handle this, deserved no trust at all.

One day, not long from now, it may be widely understood that these psychopaths in the public health profession, with their heavy-handed solutions killed ten or twenty million[91] in 2020 in the name of saving a few thousand.

Whatever other plans they have up their sleeves I am not privy to. Folks like Bill Gates say such twisted things, that if even 1% of it were true, the whole public health profession should be deported to a South Pacific atoll and left there to build exactly the society they want, far removed from the rest of us and far removed from any role of authority or public trust.

Disobeying An Unjust Order
Is Individual Nullification

For those millions of Americans, with legitimate face mask exemptions, I've created this method. When the law ceases to make room for an individual's humanity, the maker of the laws must be reminded that the law was made for man, and not man for the law.

If you don't want to go through the trouble of reminding lawmakers of such a thing, you can just individually nullify the tyrannical orders they give you.

On airplanes, at this moment in time, that means you bring a bag of beef jerky, a few sticks of gum, and fly Delta.

Maskless At Work

The idea is the same.

No different.

Be ready to walk away.

You must not work anywhere that is not moving you toward who you want to become.

In almost all scenarios, hospitals included, for a free man to be masked by his boss under the present conditions is a sign that his time in that role need come to a prompt end, or his boss need quickly rethink his decision.

Both are achieved by being ready to walk away from that job.

Maskless At School

An Arizona father writes:

Dear Mr. Stevo,

I am a public school teacher in Arizona and have been for almost 20 years.

My district is currently having a board meeting discussing our return to school Sept 8th.

The teachers who are part of the union all left comments against us returning due to metrics.

A majority of the parents are in support of kids returning to our high school where I teach. I have two kids in the local elementary school in the district and I will never ever allow my kids to be masked in a school, nor will I as a teacher. I will be resigning at the end of this quarter and homeschooling my kids, ages 5 and 3.5 due to this insane mask policy. Public school will never be the same.

Thank you for your contributions. I enjoy the free thinking that still exists.

- A.W.

A Texas school district employee writes:

Dear Mr. Stevo,

I found something of interest, referencing the Texas Association of School Boards, referencing the Education Code, in the section covering student discipline, under "aversive techniques," paragraph 7 (b) it specifically prohibits forcing students to wear a mask!

Aversive Techniques

A district or district employee or volunteer or an independent contractor of a district may not apply an aversive technique, or by authorization, order, or consent, cause an aversive technique to be applied, to a student.

"Aversive technique" means a technique or intervention that is intended to reduce the likelihood of a behavior reoccurring by intentionally inflicting on a student significant physical or emotional discomfort or pain. The term includes a technique or intervention that:...

7. Impairs the student's breathing, including any procedure that involves:

- *Applying pressure to the student's torso or neck; or*
- *Obstructing the student's airway, including placing an object in, on, or over the student's mouth or nose or placing a bag, cover, or mask over the student's face...*

- B. L.

This is taken from the *Texas Education Code* section on Prohibiting Aversive Techniques.

This Texas law[92] isn't a closed case by any means, but based on the way the law is being pointlessly thrown around by people who don't bother to read the law, especially in this "perception is reality" Covid era, why shouldn't a parent feel equally welcome to throw around the law and to do so with bluster?

Right now is a time when children deserve to see their parents fight for things that matter. Fights can be easy to pick though. All it takes is a little bit of ego. Perhaps more importantly, now is a time when children deserve to see their parents sacrifice for things that matter.

Are you willing to give up your new car, your twice yearly vacation, or other comforts of life in order to homeschool the kids? Of course those aren't the only options life offers, but now more than ever, this is a time to be willing to make major life adjustments for the betterment of your family.

Your children are watching you, and your actions speak so much louder than words. What behavior will you model in these telling moments? No one can be perfect all the time. We all make mistakes. However, it takes a certain carelessness, or even willfulness, to make all the wrong decisions in this era. Lots of people are doing just that and making all the wrong mistakes. Your kids need a parent who is going to do more than go along to get along.

Don't look at the bright side. Don't look at how much better this month is than whatever the totally messed up previous month of school looked like. Don't try to look for ways to make the revolting into the palatable. You risk normalizing it all for yourself and your children. Humans are adaptable. This can be useful in the right environments. If you put that desire for adaptability first in life, there will be no end to the amount of morals, ethics, and standards you can convince yourself to violate in order to not have to make hard decisions.

Please don't be that person. Life can be so much better than that. You can be so much more than "adaptable."

This entire book is largely about you as an individual and your interaction with the world. If this chapter applies to you, and you have children, the little ones are watching your every step.

Poet Milan Rufus[93] writes:

> Mind your kids,
> you adults.
> They are gathering your pollen,
> those little bees from God.
> They will seal it into their little bodies.
> They imitate you.
> They are the most exact living
> little mirrors of you.
>
> Their shape is from your anvils.
> They live from your bread.

One day they will be exactly like you.

So be humane to each other.

If you have children you know how little your words can mean, you know how much your actions mean. You know that this is not just a book about you and how your every action affects you. It is also a book about your children and how your seemingly smallest actions can affect them.

This is a difficult era to be a parent. The stakes are so high. I commend you for every chance you get to rise to the occasion and so willingly embrace that chance.

Nuts And Bolts

Every Face Mask Order Has Loopholes: A Michigan Case Study

You can drive a bus through Michigan's face mask exemptions.

If you and I took the teleporter to Michigan right now, we might see a lot of obediently masked people, even though Michigan has some of the loosest face mask exemptions I've ever seen.[94]

While I love to booh the villain in *The Perils of Pauline* (1914)[95] as much as the next guy does, looking at Gretchen Whitmer's face mask order, she is not a villain, and no fully functioning adult reading these pages is entitled to claim status as a damsel in distress: helpless and in need of saving.

Here are highlights of the Michigan order.

No Masks Until 5 Years Old

A lot of states and localities call for the slow suffocation of children starting at 2 years old. Not Michigan; it gives you until 5.

Those Exercising Are Exempt

The order contains an exemption if you "Are exercising when wearing a face covering would interfere with the activity."

Getting A Shave Or A Facial Or A Nose Job Is Exempt

The order contains an exemption if you "Are receiving a service for which temporary removal of the face covering is necessary."

Getting Identified At A Bank Is Exempt

The order contains an exemption if you "Are entering a business or are receiving a service and are asked to temporarily remove a face covering for identifycation purposes."

Public Speaking Is Exempt

The order contains an exemption if you "Are giving a speech for broadcast or to an audience, provided that the audience is at least six feet away from the speaker."

Pastors Preaching & Officiating Are Exempt

The order contains an exemption if you "Are officiating at a religious service." A pastor doesn't need to keep his six feet either.

The Michigan face mask order therefore appears to preference religious speech and activity over other forms of public speaking. To further drive that point home, attending church is enough to protect a person from having to wear a mask, as shown in the next section. Many states have treated churches as harshly, or more harshly, than any other place where people might gather: big box stores for instance are treated less stringently than churches in some localities.

Attending Church Exempts You

The order contains an exemption for church attendance, stating "No individual is subject to penalty under section 8 of this order for removing a mask while engaging in religious worship at a house of religious worship."

Voters Are Exempt

Those who see democracy as a god — a plentiful number of American technocrats — couldn't leave their religious activity unmentioned and unprotected in the midst of all this religious fervor.

The order contains an exemption if you "Are at a polling place for purposes of voting in an election."

Police Are Exempt

The order contains an exemption if you

> "Are actively engaged in a public safety role, including but not limited to law enforcement, firefighters, or emergency medical personnel, and where wearing a mask would seriously interfere in the performance of their public safety responsibilities."

Those Communicating With
Deaf People Are Exempt

The order contains an exemption if you "Are communicating with someone who is deaf, deafblind, or hard of hearing and where the ability to see the mouth is essential to communication."

Those Eating While Seated
At A Restaurant Are Exempt

The order contains an exemption if you "Are eating or drinking while seated at a food service establishment."

And The Biggest: The Medical Exemption

The order contains an exemption if you "Cannot medically tolerate a face covering." Some states won't even offer a medical exemption for vaccines. If you cannot medically tolerate a vaccine, you're out of luck. If you cannot medically tolerate a face mask in Michigan, Gretchen Whitmer's got your back (at least according to her order).

By the way, Michigan law allows for medical, religious, and philosophical exemptions from vaccines in daycare and preschool through 12th grade, as long as you and your child exercise those rights. This is much like the face mask orders. There are plenty of rights to be had for anyone who demands those rights be honored.

A philosophical exemption for face masks in Michigan would be amazing, but the good people of Michigan have yet to strike enough fear in the hearts of their minders for that to happen.

Not only does Michigan provide a medical exemption for face masks, it goes a step further and is very clear about how to invoke a medical exemption, going so far as to state what a business may say, so that business owners can be certain that they are neither violating the law nor bullying people.

Verbal Representation Of Medical Condition Is Enough In Michigan Under Whitmer's Order

The order advises on procedure for handling exemptions: "A business may, however, accept a customer's verbal representation that they are not wearing a face covering because they fall within a specified exception."

Verbal representation of a condition gets the job done. It says right there that it's okay for Mungo at the compliance checkpoint not to ask for a doctor's note, nor is it necessary for you to have managerial-training-program Karen at the compliance checkpoint conduct some kind of pseudo-medical intake interview at the backed-up front door.

The order invites you, as a customer, to say "I have a medical exemption," or some similar statement, such as *"I am unable to wear a face mask safely,"* but you don't even need to say that. "I am not wearing a face covering because I fall within a specified exemption. Now bugger off!" is enough under the Michigan order.

The same order invites the business manager to now accept that, perhaps saying something like

> "That's okay. Thank you for being so clear and polite about it. I know I won't get into trouble for that, now, which is something we've been worried about. Since you said it that way, I'm able to now fully comply with the order and allow you to shop in our store."

Don't Get Me Wrong, It's An Awful Order, But...

If you don't exhibit the courage to defend your rights, no matter what the order says, the fault is not on the tyrant, but on you.

In a freer place, maybe there would be less tyranny, but never in the history of man has that been a long-lasting aspect of life. Good leaders turn into awful tyrants, as soon as it's clear that no one else is guarding his grasp on power. The reason that there are periods of no tyranny in history is because a tyrant was not tolerated.

Once a tyrant is tolerated, well, you're going to get a tyrant. That's pretty much guaranteed. If a tyrant is not tolerated, you might still get a tyrant, but the tyrant won't last long.

So the choice is yours, are you going to tolerate a tyrant or not?

Don't Be One Of The Negative Smart People

Some smart people can be really negative. They don't do much with their smarts, but they can be incredibly insightful critics. Criticism is often a form of procrastination among the smart.

The missed potential is a tragedy of epic proportion. In the specific instance of the power grabs of 2020, rather than acting to stop a tyrant, some will spend their time proving how right they are.

Don't Be One Of Those Who Just Want A Story To Tell

Some people want a story to tell. If they have a choice between an easy way for them to go about their business, or if they can choose a complicated path that provides a story, they invariably opt for the distracting detour of the complicated and contorted story to be able to tell.

Some will wear the face mask to have a story, others will take their vaccine to have a story. The story is the primary goal for some, rather than the more wonderful primary goal of living free or having a joyous life.

I'll trade in a knee-slapping good story for an afternoon of pure liberty any day. Liberty is not a valid trade-off for entertainment.

People who want freedom will invoke their freedoms virtually any way they can figure it out.

Whitmer Is A Tyrant And Control Freak Who Must Be Stopped At Every Juncture

As much as this order compares favorably against many of the other face mask orders, it's worth noting that anyone who would sign an order with this level of detail explaining how one must talk in order to prevent being accosted, beaten, arrested, maimed, fined, or imprisoned, is an obvious control freak Karen.

Thank You To Those Who Carried Guns To The Capital In Spring And Summer 2020

There's tyranny in Michigan. No doubt about it. Imagine how bad it could be in Michigan if there weren't brave souls standing up and saying "No more!" demonstrating throughout 2020 that the elected officials were not the omnipotent saviors they fashioned themselves as. There are so many worse places than Michigan.

The worse places aren't worse places because they have worse elected officials. Elected officials are almost universally awful everywhere. It's because the worse places have worse leadership among the citizenry.

One day it will be resoundingly clear that the tyranny killed more than the germ. Imagine how many more would have lived through Covid in the northeast, had that tyranny not been so well tolerated.

We can't turn back time, but we can impact this moment, and we can impact our own lives, and perhaps even the future.

Do you want to bring an end to this tyranny as much as I do?

Your actions speak louder than any words.

Send Me Your Local Face Mask Order

I don't really want to see your local face mask order. I want you to *find* your local face mask order.

Because then we are one step closer to you *reading* your local face mask order. And that brings us one step closer to you *understanding* your local face mask order. And that brings us one step closer to someone *thinking* about your local face mask order.

Because I have an interesting statistic for you: *since your local face mask order has been issued, not a single person has read it and thought about it.*

I challenge you to prove me wrong.

Some may have interpreted the face mask order according to the accompanying press releases and accompanying press conferences. Some may have enforced it based on the emails the orders were attached to. Others may have been in positions of authority or enforcement and may have repeated the talking points about the orders from whatever cloud of glyphosate, mercury, and radiation that floats through the ether and that they get their information from.

But if I can get you to read it and think about it, I can get you to enact the exemptions that apply to you.

Do you know why I can get you to do that? Because you are a thinking person and anyone who encounters the lunacy of some of the ways enforcement is being handled and then compares it to the reality of what "the rules" say, is left with no choice but to laugh out loud at anyone who speaks such misinformed lunacy with such self-righteous entitlement.

Millions of people have legitimate exemptions. You may be one of them. The Gadfly Majestic is one of them. He's never worn a face mask. I estimate thousands of readers have never worn one, because hundreds have written me telling me that they never have.

It's such a joke, just not a funny one, that if you simply read the order, in 19 out of 20 situations, you won't ever have to wear a face mask again. Unless you're too gutless to insist that the order-writers and their colleagues just follow their own orders the way they are written.

I don't think many gutless people show up in whatever little corner of the world you encountered this piece of writing today. You didn't find it on the front page of Reddit or Drudge. You and I both are probably reflected by the Becky Akers commentary about Pastor Rob McCoy, who refuses to follow California lockdown orders: "If you're like me, you want your heroes full-throated and unflinching," writes Akers.[96]

I, too, like my heroes full-throated and unflinching.

For an example of a poorly executed policy, look at the face mask policy below. Until I found this face mask policy and pointed it out to a hotel manager, this is a face mask policy she was enforcing under the claim that there were absolutely no exemptions.

Does this look like an excerpt from a face mask policy with absolutely no exemptions? I'll let you be the judge:

> *"Medical exception: The Centers for Disease Control and Prevention (CDC)* [97] *and the Public Health Agency of Canada (PHAC) recognize that wearing cloth face coverings may not be possible in every situation or for some people. Consistent with CDC Mask Guidance this includes:*
>
> *"Children younger than 2 years old*
>
> *"Anyone who is unconscious, incapacitated, or otherwise unable to remove the cloth face covering without assistance*
>
> *"Please note, CDC guidelines recognize individuals outside these two categories also may be exempt from wearing face masks. Please refer to the FAQs below and additional hotel documentation for guidance on how to handle any guest request for additional exceptions.*
>
> *Hotels should work to reasonably accommodate associates and guests who may have disability-related issues wearing a mask."* [98,99]

I've now heard hundreds of stories of people exercising legitimate face mask exemptions across life by simply calling a manager beforehand and saying the words "I have a concern. *I am unable to wear a face mask safely.* May I still come by later on today?" As stated previously, that will be enough in approximately 19 out of 20 situations.

Do you know why those exemptions exist? Because we don't live in a tyrannical place yet. We live in a place where those writing these awful orders are leaving room for humans to fit into the order — if those humans claim their humanity.

And most people refuse to.

I invite you to send me your local face mask order. I will read it with pleasure. I invite you to send me the Marriott written face mask policy, the Menards written face mask policy, and your local laundromat's written face mask policy. I invite you to send me any face mask orders you'd like.

But what I'd really like is for you to read those written orders, and to use those written orders to enter into a place where you are exempt from the face mask.

I know it might be hard to even get anyone to send the written policy to you, because they don't actually know where to find it, since they've never read it. If you persist, you will get it though. And then, yes, I want you to do the work of just getting the corporate-speak-trained manager to follow their own policies and to instruct the doorknob-headed lug guarding the entrance to follow the same policies, instead of the ad hoc and widespread denigrating of people that they otherwise engage in.

All it takes is reading the order, and then getting another to do the same.

The Word "Until" — A Key Reason To Never Explain Your Face Mask Exemption

A wise man once said "You're either selling or being sold." I disagree with his dichotomous and adversarial view of life, but, indeed, there are some people who constantly look for someone to push around and for whom this approach toward life becomes self-fulfilling.

Categories To Be Mindful Of

They are the bullies, the psychopaths, the sociopaths, and the cowards.

This group moves around life looking for key indicators in those around them that communicate to the predator "I have an in," "I have a hook," or "I can get this guy."

These people are a key reason it is disadvantageous to talk about your health, disability, religion, or any other matter when trying to invoke a face mask exemption.

Don't say any more than *"I am unable to wear a face mask safely."* That's it. Leave it there. Pushy people, such as those mentioned above, will seek to push against you and traverse your boundaries. Don't get bothered by that, that's what these people do.

Tendencies Among Bullies

Bullies bully people. That's why we call them bullies. If that wasn't what got them out of bed in the morning, they wouldn't be called bullies. They live for it.

Bullies tend to flock toward positions where they can get away with bullying, perhaps even be rewarded for it. The rise of corona communism has opened up a new avenue by which bullies can bully. The face mask compliance checkpoints are one of the many new opportunities for a bully to do their thing.

And you, my friend, you are expected to do your thing. You know better than me what that is, for I don't even know you, but if you've found this piece of writing, we probably have a few things in common.

We might both believe people with face mask exemptions shouldn't be bullied into wearing them. We might both despise tyrants. We might both even believe that it is not the tyrant's fault if a person chooses to be so oppressible. Each person must stand up for himself.

There's excellent axiomatic reasons around privacy and decency. It's just none of their business. No amount of pushing or probing will change that fact and make it their business. Their pushing and probing should not shock you either, no matter how excessive or sincere it seems, because again, this is to be expected of anyone in a position that attracts bullies.

Instead of being bugged by their bullying, when at a loss for what to do, it is best to laugh out loud at them. It's never easy to tell if a person laughed out loud intentionally or accidentally. It messes with a bully's head.

With a bully, you can establish good boundaries now, or you can establish not so good boundaries later. Now will be easier. Later will be more painful.

If you don't set a firm boundary around your health and wellbeing, you're going to find yourself faced with renewed pushiness from a bully.

Cooperation And Compliance Are Not The Same

Seeing the world as a zero-sum game, a division between the haves and the have-nots, every interaction as having either a loser or a winner, an oppressor or a victim, the bully does not really comprehend the word "cooperation," but truly and deeply understands the word "compliance." Though commonly exchanged with each other as near synonyms, how incredibly different those two words are.

You see, compliance may not provide satisfaction for a bully. Compliance may signal weakness. The more outlandish the request, the more your well-intentioned "cooperation" will signal to the bully that you desire to be made into an easy victim. That's why you must never simply comply with requests from strangers who you don't have a longstanding relationship with. You do yourself a disservice.

This is the great ill behind "people pleasing." The negatives have nothing to do with making another happy. Making another happy can be a wonderful thing to do. The negatives have to do with how little regard you show for yourself in such moments.

Effective Self-Defense Against Bullies

Luckily, there are ways to protect yourself from bullies. I don't suggest you walk the path of the contrarian, by always saying "No!" In doing so you may deny yourself activity that is in your own interest. Also, being so rigid and preprogrammed makes you an easy target for the field of behaviorism called reverse psychology.

Instead, it is the 1.) Identifying of your own boundaries, 2.) Communicating of your own boundaries, and 3.) Defending of your own boundaries that should take place in such interactions.

Your actions should not be committed out of anything vaguely resembling blind obedience or blind disobedience. Doing so, especially blind obedience, makes you an easy victim for the bully. Please do no such thing at the compliance checkpoints.

Bullies Push Until They Reach Resistance

You can give the bully your entire medical history and three doctors' notes at the checkpoint. It might not matter.

The bully will push further.

You can agree to hop through the store unidirectionally and on one leg.

The bully will push further.

You can invite him home for dinner to spit in your mother's food.

The bully will push further.

Until

"We're gonna need you to wear your mask until..." is what the bully might say, in response to your sincere and fully transparent explanation of why you need an exemption.

Or they might say "Well, can't you wear your mask until...."

Until what?

Just fill in the blank based on your exemption.

"We're gonna need you to wear your mask until your heart palpitations begin and you faint."

"We're gonna need you to wear your mask until your panic attacks start and you have to rip it off your face once it's too late to bring the attack back under control."

"We're gonna need you to wear your mask until blood starts coming out of your mouth," a condition someone has recently written me about.

The Fruits Of Courage

If you don't say "No," it will get worse. The neat thing is, the courageous folks in touch with their own boundaries are rewarded in this situation. They bring the conflict to a head quickly. They consequently get it resolved relatively painlessly and easily.

"I am unable to wear a face mask safely," quickly draws a boundary and communicates what is needed.

If you don't draw a boundary, the bully will wrap you in tricks to take advantage of you and do his best to ruin the most special things about you, anything that you lay bare for that bully.

It's just what bullies do.

Clear And Impenetrable Boundaries Are Healthy And Protective Of That Which Is Special

That's one way promiscuity is so harmful. Important human emotions are laid bare before people who do not deserve the trust. Pearls before swine. The odds are not in favor of those who allow intimacy to be pushed into the door of a relationship before the trust necessary to make it a safe environment is earned.

I don't know what your mask-related health concerns are. It's none of my business. And it's definitely not the business of the compliance checker at the door.

Do yourself a favor, and keep your private matters to yourself.

Do yourself a favor and never again wear a face mask that you are exempt from wearing.

Name Dropping

Being able to comfortably name the manager of the site is probably the most helpful detail at any compliance checkpoint.

The words "Michelle said it was okay," or "I spoke to Trevor and got his approval," erases almost all opposition immediately. Knowing the first name of the supervisor you spoke to is key and being able to easily reference them and ask for them in all future conversations makes life far easier.

If a conversation with a site manager is ending without you having this detail, "My name is Allan. What was your name again?" should quickly get it for you.

That information should then immediately be stored in a way commensurate to how you would store all your most important keys to all your most important doors.

It is a password. It is a master key. It is a calming statement of reassurance and belonging to even the most aggressive gatekeepers. A few scribbles on a piece of paper can easily make your life ten times easier.

How To Get A Doctor's Note

This topic could be a book unto itself, elaborating on what freedom looks like in healthcare.

As a patient are you an individual? The thousands-of years-long trend in medicine says unequivocally that you are an individual. The century-and-a-half field of public health exists precisely with the intent of making you not an individual. It is collectivism or communitarianism applied to medicine.

The two should naturally behave like oil and water and have nothing to do with each other, in the absence of some unnatural force imposing an emulsion upon them.

Some people seek to make everything political and ultimately divisive. This divisiveness is easy to accomplish once a field of inquiry has been politicized.

Medicine should be a practice between doctor and patient, full of well-founded scientific hypotheses and informed trial and error, according to their comfort levels.

It generally is not that. Medicine has become groupthink. It is risk avoidance. It is seeing a patient as a statistic or probability and not an individual.

The public health approach and the medical approach are very different approaches.

This is the world we live in, one of politicized, polarized, collectivist medicine.

The further you can get from that, the more likely you are to get medical care tailor made for you, which is what the gold standard of medical care has always been.

Far from that is something called the "standard of care," which sounds similar, but is merely a good way for a doctor to try to avoid a lawsuit, and to not have to think too hard or care too much.

It is a truly awful concept, befitting a healthcare system that views itself more like a factory than a doctor's office.

The collectivist and communitarian collaborators of the public health community are the modern technocrat. There is so much overlap between these two groups that it is challenging to see where one begins and the other ends. Their speech and mannerisms can consequently be nearly identical. They are easy to spot.

The technocrat takes modern hospitals and applies the principles of highly organized factory floors to them.

A few principles that work in one area of life can be useful in other areas of life. There is no doubt about that, but there is a limit to how close to a factory one can get before a patient is no longer seen as a patient, a human being, an individual, an inviolable creation of God, and is instead seen as a widget upon which a process is performed with predictable input and output.

The whole notion is contrary to what medicine is. It is contrary to what a human is. It is contrary to what a patient is.

Factories depend on commodities: predictable inputs, in order to achieve predictable outputs. Oil can be treated as a commodity. It can have certain properties. The commodity known as West Texas Intermediate[100] is: described to be "light" and "sweet."

West Texas Intermediate shipments into the Cushing storage hub must meet the following specifications: 0.42% or less sulphur by weight, between 37 and 42° specific gravity on the API scale, less than 1% BSW (sediment, water, and other impurities), a pour point no greater than 50°F, Micro Carbon Residue less than 2.40% by weight, Total Acid Number less than 0.28 mg KOH/g, less than 8 ppm nickel by weight, and less than 15 ppm vanadium by weight.

This categorization and commoditization process is easy to do with some objects. Medicine evolved precisely because this was not possible to do with humans.

The industrial era, which has figured out how to commoditize many aspects of nature — often with considerable failure, as the process is so over applied — is constantly pushing for ways to figure out how to fit individual humans into a predictable box with a predictable input and output.

This way of thinking is anti-human and contrary to reality. Any time this thinking exists, it deserves recognition and isolation as a mere thought exercise on efficiency.

It is not theology. It is not philosophy. It is not a study of human action. It is not able to identify grand, life-improving truths. It is a pursuit of single-digit percentage achievements, often infinitesimal fractions of achievements and only when measured with some very fuzzy math.

That minor achievement comes at the cost of big aims.

American attorney Ralph Nader made a name for himself by catching the auto makers cutting corners on safety in order to save a few dollars. If they were likely to lose more in lawsuits from not using a safety feature than they saved by not using a safety feature, then they would include the feature.

Nader used this equation against the auto manufacturers by inspiring so many lawsuits, that safety suddenly became a top priority for auto manufacturers.

It's debatable how much Nader's actions benefitted individual consumers, but the impact he had upon the American auto industry is undeniably monumental.

Nader and other attorneys like him, helped to inspire a safety obsessed, risk-averse, and far more collectivist version of the United States. Consequently, he helped to drive the thinking that brought the Covid scare of 2020.

A great cultural shift took place. By majoring in minor things, American popular culture has lost the ability to turn out great music and great cars and has come to focus on a great deal of impotence, frivolity, and infinitesimal benefit.

Can one possibly forgive Ford Motor Company for avoiding change to save a few bucks, even if it means greater and predictable loss of life? Sure. That's what companies exist to do: please consumers cheaply. If you want a different car that isn't built based on that principle, you go elsewhere.

But what if someone stopped you from going elsewhere? What if that was all you could get? What if someone stopped everyone who provided an alternative to Ford from even existing? This is what we find in the healthcare system: corporate, profit-cutting efficiency. It is brilliant for some patients, especially those who want to have a predictable process and want to be treated as a predictable input and output, who want to be treated as a commodity effectively on the factory floor.

It is horrible for those who want something different: a Porsche, a Rolls Royce, a bicycle, a motorcycle, a golf cart, a row boat, or a parachute. What if that was what you wanted, but all you could get was a 1975 Ford Pinto. That's what the medical system increasingly offers: a one-size-fits-all approach.

They call it "standard of care." Sure, there are lots of options, but you still have a 1975 Ford Pinto when all is said and done.

State and federal regulators, medical boards, lobbyists, pharmaceutical companies, hospitals, and various other trade organizations and special interest groups work very hard and spend massive budgets making sure the 1975 Ford Pinto is all you can get out of healthcare.

Year-by-year, their hold on that system appears to magnify and year-by-year more people who demand better squeeze out of that system, sometimes even finding themselves in a situation where they must decide to either break the law or submit to 1975 Ford Pinto style healthcare. The exploding 1975 Ford Pinto was a regrettable car from the era when "contempt for the customer" ruled automotive manufacturing.

This is where we find ourselves in 2020 with the latest one-size-fits-all approach to medicine: the face mask.

"If you don't want to wear a face mask, just go get a doctor's note," is a common answer. It's an awful answer though in such an increasingly uniform and controlled medical system.

The best answer to this is to pushback and refuse to seek a doctor's note, especially for an ongoing condition that you have not needed to seek treatment in years, if ever, and for which you have no relationship with a doctor.

You will be hard pressed to find a doctor willing to write you a note for a decade-old condition that he has never treated you for. The era is just too political and the risk to the doctor too great.

Some people, having pushed back, are left in a corner and really have determined that their only course of action is that they need to get a doctor's note. Never is there only one course of action. There are always more options. I strongly recommend you consider all options.

Here are a few thoughts that have been useful for others, in obtaining a doctor's note.

Step 1: Relationship

If you have done the hard work and have an ongoing relationship with a doctor who views your healthcare as an individual matter, the way you do, and assesses the whole person, then you are in a good position. If not, you are in a good position to start finding that doctor now. Unless you plan to have a very short rest of your life, you would be foolish to think the politicization of your healthcare stops with face masks. You are going to need an ally who sees you as an individual human and not a commodity at the sprocket factory.

Step 2: It's A Numbers Game

The more you try, the more you have a chance at getting what you want, especially when you analyze and refine your technique along the way.

Step 3: Cold Calling

Sometimes the best way to learn what is happening in the world is to pick up the phone and ask people for what you want. Do that enough and you will learn a lot along the way and eventually refine your process to get exactly who you need.

Step 4: Referrals

Tap your network. A doctor who knows someone who knows you may be more likely to help you than a stranger, especially given the fact that states employ "testers," in all manner of industries, to entrap a practitioner in an industry.

Step 5: Outside The Box

An OD, psychologist, naturopath, a popular figure, alternative health practitioner, an academic, or a researcher with an MD might all be possible professionals who can help you. Get a note from anyone you trust and put the onus on the other party to refute the validity of such a note. Some compliance enforcers won't bother and will consider the box checked with their receipt of a note.

Step 6: Resources

If you are able to go beyond your in-network provider, that may help. If you can pay cash, that may help. You might even be able to negotiate for this specialized service. In the United States, doctors who accept Medicare

are not, by law, able to negotiate payments with other patients. To the best of my understanding, those who do not accept Medicare may negotiate service on a patient-by-patient basis.

Step 7: Doctors Who Already See Beyond The Medical Establishment

Doctors who already see beyond the medical establishment on one topic may be more open to doing the same on this topic. This might include doctors who work with experimental treatments, emotional support animals, vaccine injury, with toxicity from industrial metals, or many other areas of specialization that require a doctor to have a view that is beyond the medical establishment.

Step 8: Don't Give Up

If this is important to you, it will happen. But again, I consider this search for a doctor a rather ineffective way to get around a bad mask order. The upside is that it helps you find a doctor for the future who can be a lifelong ally to you as an individual patient seeking individualized care.

How To Find A Lawyer

Over the past month of advocating for civil disobedience against the corona ban, I've received many requests on how a person goes about suing the government.

A wonderful and fitting article about being civilly disobedient ran at the American Institute for Economic Research entitled "Why Aren't Americans Suing Their Way Out Of Lockdown?"[101]

That article, by Robert E. Wright, presents a legal framework for why more lawsuits should take place. Below, I'm going to offer a framework for HOW to make that happen.

If the courts were inundated with 30 million lawsuits tomorrow, it would be a great thing. I once had the joy of suing the government in a manner similar to this one. Alternately, if even one key test case is brought before the courts successfully, as Wright describes in his piece, it could have a tremendous impact that ripples through the country.

I'm not deluding myself into thinking that the government judiciary will free America from government tyranny, but once in a while they require a tyrant to explain himself, allow a citizen to redress grievances, and occasionally act as a tool to help right wrongs.

If you think you have been harmed by the corona bans, lockdowns, mandatory masking, or any other aspect of the governmental response to corona, below are some first steps that can be taken to help set a lawsuit into motion.

Step 1: Decide: Pro Se, Public Interest & Pro Bono, Or Your Own Private Attorney

"Pro se" means you represent yourself. A lot of people have a lot of fun doing that. You learn a lot about the process. Though I think it's a great education, I'm not convinced it is right for this pressing, emergency topic.

If you decide you'd like to do this pro se, the rest of the chapter is irrelevant, so please get to work on that and Godspeed. May you have the greatest of success. For the rest of you, I'll continue.

Public interest lawyers seek cases that have a benefit that goes beyond just one person. They tend to seek a grave government injustice that needs addressing and overturning. Sometimes they work free of charge to their client, or "pro bono." I believe on this topic, there are many lawyers out there who will take a case pro bono if asked.

Many more attorneys will take this case for money. There may be a lower level of philosophical commitment in that situation and a higher level of economic commitment.

I would suggest starting by seeking a pro bono attorney and keeping track of the paid attorneys you encounter along the way with a noted interest in your specific case, in case you decide to reach back out to them and fund the case yourself.

Step 2: Keep Organized

Simple spreadsheets are good for this. Pads of paper are useful, but not great, because URLs can be long. You'll want columns for the lawyer's name, URL, phone number, dates you've reached out, and responses.

Everything you learn during your search should end up in your spreadsheet, because having everything in one place will make the succeeding steps easier.

Step 3: Identify Potential Lawyers

During this next step, you are aiming to find a broad selection of lawyers. Similar to the process of brainstorming, you are adding anyone who might take the case to your list, regardless of whatever downsides there might be to working with them. The longer the list made in this step, the better.

Are There Authors Or Legal Theorists You Like?

If you have a favorite author on this topic who has a law degree, chances are he knows other lawyers with a passion for this topic. Reach out. Ask for a referral.

Though the list is from 2011, Walter Block compiled a fantastic, exhaustive list of libertarian legal theorists, found in the appendix of this book, that can serve as a useful reference.

Constitutional lawyer Robert Barnes has been active in the media on Covid-19 overreach. His firm may take an interest in representing you. Based on conversations with clients of his, that firm takes cases in a number of states.

Are There Cases You Have Followed?

There might be notable public interest cases you've heard of. They may have taken place a few years back. See if you can find the lawyers who were involved with those cases. There could be a lawyer whose work you respect and who knows how to use the courts to gets things done. Reach out.

Tap Your Network

You likely know lawyers personally. Tell them what you plan to do, ask them if they know anyone who might be interested. Send them a version of your letter from the step below.

If you feel like a direct request for them to represent you is too bold, you can ask "Do you happen to know a lawyer who could represent me in a lawsuit against the lockdown orders?" or "Might you be able to refer me to a lawyer who could represent me in a lawsuit against the lockdown orders?"

You likely know non-lawyers who know lawyers. Check with them too.

People who share your passion about this topic are probably going to be better to reach out to than those who have been on Next Door snitching on neighbors and calling for 18-month rolling lockdowns.

Try to make sure that anyone you reach out to goes into your spreadsheet. Using your network is probably forty to fifty times more effective, for the average person, than reaching out cold, but you can find available lawyers through a cold process as well.

Examples Of Public Interest Lawyers Who May Take An Interest In Your Corona Case

Institute for Justice has at least one member of their staff who has taken an interest in the topic of corona bans and invites people to submit details, like the letter above to their "Report Abuse" section of their website, which is the page dedicated to asking IJ for legal assistance on a matter.

The Thomas More Law Center focuses on family values, life, religious freedom, and calls itself "the Christian response to the ACLU."

Southeastern Legal Foundation is a public interest law firm and policy center that advocates for limited government, individual liberty, and free enterprise.

Pacific Justice Institute advocates for the defense of religious freedom, parental rights, and other civil liberties.

The Freedom of Conscience Defense Fund seeks to make sure cases get heard not only at the local level, but also at the appellate level, a useful niche for helping to combat bad policy.

Landmark Legal Foundation is a national non-profit law firm preserving constitutional values such as limited government, separation of powers, and federalism.

American Civil Liberties Union has a network of staffed offices in every state, Washington DC, and Puerto Rico. Their local affiliates can be contacted directly to see if a case is of interest.

The ACLU has at least one lawsuit seeking to overturn a corona ban. Rather than a central office determining what cases they will take, if you contact your local ACLU chapter, you can find out if they would 1.) take your case or 2.) send a referral out to their referral network.

Judicial Watch mainly uses litigation to help uncover government malfeasance. In preparation for this writing, they notified me by phone that they were not presently interested in this topic.

The James Madison Center exists to protect free expression.

The First Amendment Lawyers Association will distribute your request to their membership from their contact page.

Liberty Counsel filed a lawsuit on behalf of Maryville Baptist Church in Louisville and its pastor Jack Roberts against Kentucky Gov. Andy Beshear — for the singling out of his church in a particularly brutal enforcement of the corona lockdown, as other businesses nearby had full parking lots and few restrictions. Liberty Counsel is currently representing pastors in more than 30 states.

The Alliance for Defending Freedom had a recent victory in Kansas with a federal judge ruling to protect churches from a corona ban and Tyson Langhofer of the organization pointing out "Public safety is important, but so is following the Constitution."

The Center for American Liberty, is a legal advocacy organization, that is fighting the California lockdown orders on several fronts, including filing a lawsuit against Gov. Gavin Newsom last week for prohibiting in-person church services, as well as representing an organizer of a San Diego protest against the lockdown.

In Ohio, **1851 Center for Constitutional Law**, is bringing a lawsuit on behalf of bridal shop owner Tanya Rutner Hartman, against Ohio Health Director Dr. Amy Acton In US District Court, challenging the constitutionality of ordering her business closed for being non-essential.

The 1851 Center is "A non-profit, non-partisan law firm dedicated to protecting the constitutional rights of Ohioans from government." The state you live in may have a similar state-specific organization.

Arizona's **Goldwater Institute** takes on litigation in Arizona and across the country and has a network of lawyers, the American Freedom Network, for cases that the Goldwater Institute does not take on.

If you are at a loss in identifying a state specific organization, the **State Policy Network** Membership Directory, may be a good starting place. In that directory, almost every organization designates a contact person as well as listing an email and phone number for reaching them.

Keep in mind that not all members show a strong interest in litigating and, naturally, not all organizations that will take an interest in this topic are included in their membership list. Many other organizations exist, this is merely a subset.

Tap THEIR Referral Network

Every group on the list above has attorneys in their orbit who care deeply about the topics that those groups focus on.

If they don't have someone on staff who wants to work with you, they may be willing to send out information about your request to their network. That email to the network can be very effective in finding a lawyer. Keep this in mind.

If in response to a referral request, they say "Contact your local bar association," that is lawyer speak for "Take a hike, we're not interested." Don't take that personally.

"Cold Call" Lawyers

Open a search engine, enter your jurisdiction and "public interest law" and go from there. You will find many options and will likely get a response from anywhere between 1-out-of-10 and 1-out-of-50 lawyers who you reach out to.

Some will have email addresses that you can easily find, while others will be more likely to have contact forms that go directly to their intake coordinator.

Step 4: Create A Form Letter That Says Enough, But Not Too Much

Until a lawyer represents you, there's no need to tell them your deepest secrets on this topic. Keep the form letter short and to the point: you are seeking representation, you see clear precedent, are they interested?

If you'd like a template, something like this might work:

Dear First Name Last Name,

I'm looking for a pro bono attorney to represent me on a public interest case regarding the Covid-19 order in my state, (insert state).

The New York Supreme Court has previously ruled against widespread quarantines, establishing a clear precedent in the 1856 New York Supreme Court case *The People vs. Peter W. Roff*, mentioned by a think-tank fellow recently in this linked article. I wonder if there may be other meaningful precedent on this topic.

Would you be willing to represent me?

If you would not, can you recommend someone who might want to?

Thank you.

First Name Last Name
City, State
Email address

Step 5: Follow Through

For some people, though quite unlikely, it will take just one hour of work to identify an eager lawyer, for others it may take ten hours of work.

In either case, you can get most of that work done today. You can sit down, and decide that by the three-hour mark, you will have sent 10 emails out to lawyers. In some situations, you might not follow up for a week.

But in this situation, as you find every minute and every inch of your personal liberty important to you, you resolve that you will give them two days to respond and will go right down that list with a follow-up email 48 hours from now.

Step 6: Speak Ideally To A Few Lawyers

Since time is of the essence, I recognize why it may not make sense to speak to a few lawyers, but to instead go with the first excited lawyer you encounter.

Every lawyer is going to have a different take on your case. You want to take notes about everything a lawyer says to you about the case, so that you can bounce ideas off others you speak to.

Most cases don't see the light of day because it is so genuinely difficult to find representation. Many legitimate cases go unheard. It really is a matter of you keeping organized and diligently following through.

The corona bans are illegal and unconstitutional. They are executive and bureaucratic over-reach. Many lawyers out there will happily take on a case like yours.

<u>Step 7</u>: Choose A Lawyer

Read online reviews. Ask the prospective lawyer questions. This lawyer is doing you a favor – without them there is no case. But you are also doing them a favor – without you there is no case.

So you are going to want someone who you think will work well with you and who will be a good teammate. In all likelihood, they will want you to not participate in much and to mostly be a name on a document.

Will you want regular check-ins? Will you want to see the legal drafts and be able to comment? What do they need from you to make this a success? What is their motivation for getting involved? Are they committed to the idea? Are they diligent? Are they knowledgeable about this specific topic? Do they have a record of past successes? Do they have past clients you can call, from both successful and unsuccessful cases?

Step 8: Focus On Your Next Instance Of Civil Disobedience

Your lawyer is now going to do almost all the work. It is time for you to get out there and find another front to push on.

The most important thing is that you get the ball rolling today.

Good luck with this.

What If They Tell Me To Wear Other PPE?

There are lots of different items called personal protective equipment (PPE).

Most of it doesn't do much to protect from Covid. In CDC labs where bio-weapons are studied, the PPE is far more significant than a surgical mask, a neck gaiter, or an N95 mask.

Dozens of times, I've been told "Well, can't you just cover your nose with a Kleenex, to make others feel more comfortable?" or "Can't you just hold a hand up to your mouth so other customers can feel more at ease?" or "Our policy states that anyone not wearing a face mask must cover up with a face shield."

The argument for alternative PPE is preposterous and lays bare the fact that so little of this has anything to do with science or safety. It has a lot to do with complacency, control, community, and feelings. That's just not spoken of very honestly. The word "science" is used to talk about that which is not scientific.

To use a word to mean the opposite of what it actually means is also known as a lie.

As pointed out earlier, I do not accept the alternate PPE suggestions as a legitimate response to a face mask exemption:

In a medical or dental setting, they are used to all kinds of personal protective equipment (PPE), so they might say that it's fine to not wear a face mask, but that you must wear some other type of PPE, such as a face shield.

To this, introduction of a new form of PPE, you can now start the whole process over again. You may be one of the many millions who cannot safely wear a face shield either. In the example of a face shield, you can again respond "In your policy, what are your face shield exemptions?"

After they send you the exemptions, you can have a look to see if you fit the exemptions, and state "I am unable to wear a face shield safely. Can you make the proper arrangements for me to come in?"

Whatever type of exotic PPE that is suggested to you, I recommend the same process: "What are the exemptions in your policy around that?" followed by "I am unable to wear it safely," provided that applies to you. It applies to many millions.

Though it may be appealing to leap at the fact that a face shield worn on its own is not efficacious, and to ridicule the person and their suggestion, I encourage you to leave that topic alone. The more a person suggests various alternate PPE for you to wear, rather than just *dropping the whole subject and honoring your requested exemption, the more it becomes clear that it's about emotion, optics, and control rather than science, health, and safety. Repeated suggestions like that speak volumes and call into question whether this is really someone who you want making decisions with you about your health.*

People may suffer all the same problems from the alternate options and require an exemption from them as well. If you have a legitimate exemption to a face mask, you may also have a legitimate exemption to all other forms of PPE.

The same method works just as well on other PPE as it does on face masks.

When asked to wear alternate PPE, I hope you will take an extra critical moment to contemplate what kind of person you are likely speaking to, who has little intent to honor your exemption and who has somehow concluded that a "Kleenex held near the face," or a plastic face shield has enough proven efficacy to haggle over it at this moment. What is it really about to someone like that? Why would you want to be anywhere near such a person?

Whether it is lack of intellectual wherewithal or sinister intent to control another, that person in a position of authority does not deserve such a position.

Sometimes it takes moments like these to determine how unfit a person is for the leadership role he is in.

Email Or Phone?

Email and phone each have advantages. Phone allows for more flexible and direct interaction, easier reading of social cues, greater ability to build rapport or to exercise already built rapport.

Having made more than 100,000 cold calls in 2012 for my preferred presidential candidate and having helped build, staff, train, or manage phone banks making many millions more calls, phone is by far my preferred method between the two options, and I believe it is in almost all situations the better option for most people.

If you are worried about not being ready to answer a question on the spot, then email may be the way to go since it will give you a little extra time to think over your response and to say what you need to. Email also has the advantage of helping you create a record. In some situations, having a record can be very helpful in the preparation of legal action, but the idea of pulling a "gotcha" on someone in court over face masks is so far from my mind.

I'm just trying to help people communicate better and cooperate better in this supremely emotional and divisive era and topic.

I don't think even one time in my life that I have believed an email got the point across better than a phone call. Covid is the first time in my life that I've ever seen a phone call be more effective than a face-to-face conver-

sation. That is only because some people are so morti-
fied by the sight of an unmasked face that they can't get
beyond the sight well enough to concentrate on the
request being made.

Conditions

Specific Conditions
That May Exempt You

In the following pages The Lesson is applied repetitively to the following conditions:

Asthma, surgeries, heart conditions, COPD, migraines, panic attacks, claustrophobia, psychological conditions, multiple sclerosis, auto-immune disorder, cancer, chronic lung ailments, terminal heart conditions, dyspnea, angina, cephalalgia, internal physical deformations from injuries, genetic abnormalities, and breathing.

This promises to be a repetitive section of *Face Masks In One Lesson,* because very little new information is needed for any single condition. Moreover, no one but you and a trusted healthcare provider approved by you, have any business dictating what is in your best interest health-wise.

That trusted healthcare provider is no dictator at all, but merely an advisor welcome to share his insight with you in exchange for some fiduciary compensation and the honor of your momentary respect and consideration.

Please, do not even for one minute, and for any reason, ever again feel compelled by another to wear a face mask that may be unsafe for you to wear.

Despite your obvious recognition that such a condition is impactful to you, it is my firm belief that no one at a compliance checkpoint is entitled to demand that you explain any condition to them.

"I am unable to wear a face mask safely," need be all you tell a face mask compliance checker.

Asthma

With a mere wiggle of an inhaler to a compliance checker, a person can easily get past many face mask checkpoints. The existence of inhalers and the memory of seeing sudden, scary asthma attacks has been witnessed by many.

Asthma at every diagnosable stage can cause a person to have difficulty wearing a face mask safely.

Asthma, being so poorly understood in the general population, it is my suggestion that you not mention asthma at a compliance checkpoint. You may appear perfectly healthy to the untrained eye.

This does not change the fact that shortly after putting on a face mask, you may find yourself in discomfort. It's not worth it.

"I am unable to wear a face mask safely," will get the job done. No need to mention any more at a checkpoint if this describes your exemption.

The choice to be masked or not must be left up to you, not some far off paper pusher who doesn't even know you, let alone examined you, taken your history, and tried to understand you as an individual with a unique set of wants and needs.

Surgeries

Among my neighbors who I regularly see, two have had surgery over the past few months. They did not advertise the surgery beforehand. They just disappeared for a time (2-3 weeks) and upon their return to the walking path we frequent, they looked just as they had before: the same weight, the same level of fitness, and the same jovial voices. Only later did I learn from each of them that they had surgeries and were undergoing further treatment.

Recovering from surgery, at every stage, can cause a person to have difficulty wearing a face mask safely.

Surgeries, being so poorly understood in the general population, it is my suggestion that you not mention surgeries at a compliance checkpoint. You may appear perfectly healthy to the untrained eye.

This does not change the fact that shortly after putting on a face mask, you may find yourself in discomfort. It's not worth it.

"I am unable to wear a face mask safely," will get the job done. No need to mention any more at a checkpoint if this describes your exemption.

The choice to be masked or not must be left up to you, not some far off paper pusher who doesn't even know you, let alone examined you, taken your history, and tried to understand you as an individual with a unique set of wants and needs.

Heart Conditions

Heart conditions at every diagnosable stage can cause a person to have difficulty wearing a face mask safely.

Heart conditions, being so poorly understood in the general population, it is my suggestion that you not mention heart conditions at a compliance checkpoint. You may appear perfectly healthy to the untrained eye.

This does not change the fact that shortly after putting on a face mask, you may find yourself in discomfort. It's not worth it.

"I am unable to wear a face mask safely," will get the job done. No need to mention any more at a checkpoint if this describes your exemption.

The choice to be masked or not must be left up to you, not some far off paper pusher who doesn't even know you, let alone examined you, taken your history, and tried to understand you as an individual with a unique set of wants and needs.

COPD

COPD at every diagnosable stage can cause a person to have difficulty wearing a face mask safely.

COPD, being so poorly understood in the general population, it is my suggestion that you not mention COPD at a compliance checkpoint. You may appear perfectly healthy to the untrained eye.

This does not change the fact that shortly after putting on a face mask, you may find yourself in discomfort. It's not worth it.

"I am unable to wear a face mask safely," will get the job done. No need to mention any more at a check-point if this describes your exemption.

The choice to be masked or not must be left up to you, not some far off paper pusher who doesn't even know you, let alone examined you, taken your history, and tried to understand you as an individual with a unique set of wants and needs.

Migraines

Migraines at every diagnosable stage can cause a person to have difficulty wearing a face mask safely.

Migraines, being so poorly understood in the general population, it is my suggestion that you not mention migraines at a compliance checkpoint. You may appear perfectly healthy to the untrained eye.

This does not change the fact that shortly after putting on a face mask, you may find yourself in discomfort. It's not worth it.

"I am unable to wear a face mask safely," will get the job done. No need to mention any more at a checkpoint if this describes your exemption.

The choice to be masked or not must be left up to you, not some far off paper pusher who doesn't even know you, let alone examined you, taken your history, and tried to understand you as an individual with a unique set of wants and needs.

Panic Attacks

Panic attacks at every diagnosable stage can cause a person to have difficulty wearing a face mask safely.

Panic attacks, being so poorly understood in the general population, it is my suggestion that you not mention panic attacks at a compliance checkpoint. You may appear perfectly healthy to the untrained eye.

This does not change the fact that shortly after putting on a face mask, you may find yourself in discomfort. It's not worth it.

"I am unable to wear a face mask safely," will get the job done. No need to mention any more at a checkpoint if this describes your exemption.

The choice to be masked or not must be left up to you, not some far off paper pusher who doesn't even know you, let alone examined you, taken your history, and tried to understand you as an individual with a unique set of wants and needs.

Claustrophobia

Claustrophobia at every diagnosable stage can cause a person to have difficulty wearing a face mask safely.

Claustrophobia, being so poorly understood in the general population, it is my suggestion that you not mention claustrophobia at a compliance checkpoint. You may appear perfectly healthy to the untrained eye.

This does not change the fact that shortly after putting on a face mask, you may find yourself in discomfort. It's not worth it.

"I am unable to wear a face mask safely," will get the job done. No need to mention any more at a checkpoint if this describes your exemption.

The choice to be masked or not must be left up to you, not some far off paper pusher who doesn't even know you, let alone examined you, taken your history, and tried to understand you as an individual with a unique set of wants and needs.

Psychological Conditions

Psychological conditions at every diagnosable stage can cause a person to have difficulty wearing a face mask safely.

Psychological conditions, being so poorly understood in the general population, it is my suggestion that you not mention psychological conditions at a compliance checkpoint. You may appear perfectly healthy to the untrained eye.

This does not change the fact that shortly after putting on a face mask, you may find yourself in discomfort. It's not worth it.

"I am unable to wear a face mask safely," will get the job done. No need to mention any more at a checkpoint if this describes your exemption.

The choice to be masked or not must be left up to you, not some far off paper pusher who doesn't even know you, let alone examined you, taken your history, and tried to understand you as an individual with a unique set of wants and needs.

Multiple Sclerosis

Multiple sclerosis at every diagnosable stage can cause a person to have difficulty wearing a face mask safely.

Multiple sclerosis, being so poorly understood in the general population, it is my suggestion that you not mention multiple sclerosis at a compliance checkpoint. You may appear perfectly healthy to the untrained eye.

This does not change the fact that shortly after putting on a face mask, you may find yourself in discomfort. It's not worth it.

"I am unable to wear a face mask safely," will get the job done. No need to mention any more at a checkpoint if this describes your exemption.

The choice to be masked or not must be left up to you, not some far off paper pusher who doesn't even know you, let alone examined you, taken your history, and tried to understand you as an individual with a unique set of wants and needs.

Auto-Immune Disorders

Auto-immune disorders at every diagnosable stage can cause a person to have difficulty wearing a face mask safely.

Auto-immune disorders, being so poorly understood in the general population, it is my suggestion that you not mention auto-immune disorders at a compliance checkpoint. You may appear perfectly healthy to the untrained eye.

This does not change the fact that shortly after putting on a face mask, you may find yourself in discomfort. It's not worth it.

"I am unable to wear a face mask safely," will get the job done. No need to mention any more at a checkpoint if this describes your exemption.

The choice to be masked or not must be left up to you, not some far off paper pusher who doesn't even know you, let alone examined you, taken your history, and tried to understand you as an individual with a unique set of wants and needs.

Cancer

Cancer at every diagnosable stage can cause a person to have difficulty wearing a face mask safely.

Cancer, being so poorly understood in the general population, it is my suggestion that you not mention cancer at a compliance checkpoint. You may appear perfectly healthy to the untrained eye.

This does not change the fact that shortly after putting on a face mask, you may find yourself in discomfort. It's not worth it.

"I am unable to wear a face mask safely," will get the job done. No need to mention any more at a checkpoint if this describes your exemption.

The choice to be masked or not must be left up to you, not some far off paper pusher who doesn't even know you, let alone examined you, taken your history, and tried to understand you as an individual with a unique set of wants and needs.

Chronic Lung Ailments

Chronic lung ailments at every diagnosable stage can cause a person to have difficulty wearing a face mask safely.

Chronic lung ailments, being so poorly understood in the general population, it is my suggestion that you not mention chronic lung ailments at a compliance check-point. You may appear perfectly healthy to the un-trained eye.

This does not change the fact that shortly after putting on a face mask, you may find yourself in discomfort. It's not worth it.

"I am unable to wear a face mask safely," will get the job done. No need to mention any more at a check-point if this describes your exemption.

The choice to be masked or not must be left up to you, not some far off paper pusher who doesn't even know you, let alone examined you, taken your history, and tried to understand you as an individual with a unique set of wants and needs.

Dyspnea (Shortness Of Breath)

Dyspnea at every diagnosable stage can cause a person to have difficulty wearing a face mask safely.

Dyspnea, being so poorly understood in the general population, it is my suggestion that you not mention dyspnea at a compliance checkpoint. You may appear perfectly healthy to the untrained eye.

This does not change the fact that shortly after putting on a face mask, you may find yourself in discomfort. It's not worth it.

"I am unable to wear a face mask safely," will get the job done. No need to mention any more at a checkpoint if this describes your exemption.

The choice to be masked or not must be left up to you, not some far off paper pusher who doesn't even know you, let alone examined you, taken your history, and tried to understand you as an individual with a unique set of wants and needs.

Angina (Chest Pains)

Angina at every diagnosable stage can cause a person to have difficulty wearing a face mask safely.

Angina, being so poorly understood in the general population, it is my suggestion that you not mention angina at a compliance checkpoint. You may appear perfectly healthy to the untrained eye.

This does not change the fact that shortly after putting on a face mask, you may find yourself in discomfort. It's not worth it.

"I am unable to wear a face mask safely," will get the job done. No need to mention any more at a checkpoint if this describes your exemption.

The choice to be masked or not must be left up to you, not some far off paper pusher who doesn't even know you, let alone examined you, taken your history, and tried to understand you as an individual with a unique set of wants and needs.

Cephalalgia (Headaches)

Cephalalgia at every diagnosable stage can cause a person to have difficulty wearing a face mask safely.

Cephalalgia, being so poorly understood in the general population, it is my suggestion that you not mention cephalalgia at a compliance checkpoint. You may appear perfectly healthy to the untrained eye.

This does not change the fact that shortly after putting on a face mask, you may find yourself in discomfort. It's not worth it.

"I am unable to wear a face mask safely," will get the job done. No need to mention any more at a checkpoint if this describes your exemption.

The choice to be masked or not must be left up to you, not some far off paper pusher who doesn't even know you, let alone examined you, taken your history, and tried to understand you as an individual with a unique set of wants and needs.

Internal Physical Deformations From Injuries

Internal physical deformations from injuries at every diagnosable stage can cause a person to have difficulty wearing a face mask safely.

Internal physical deformations from injuries, being so poorly understood in the general population, it is my suggestion that you not mention internal physical deformations from injuries at a compliance checkpoint. You may appear perfectly healthy to the untrained eye.

This does not change the fact that shortly after putting on a face mask, you may find yourself in discomfort. It's not worth it.

"I am unable to wear a face mask safely," will get the job done. No need to mention any more at a checkpoint if this describes your exemption.

The choice to be masked or not must be left up to you, not some far off paper pusher who doesn't even know you, let alone examined you, taken your history, and tried to understand you as an individual with a unique set of wants and needs.

Genetic Abnormalities

Genetic abnormalities at every diagnosable stage can cause a person to have difficulty wearing a face mask safely.

Genetic abnormalities, being so poorly understood in the general population, it is my suggestion that you not mention genetic abnormalities at a compliance check-point. You may appear perfectly healthy to the un-trained eye.

This does not change the fact that shortly after putting on a face mask, you may find yourself in discomfort. It's not worth it.

"I am unable to wear a face mask safely," will get the job done. No need to mention any more at a check-point if this describes your exemption.

The choice to be masked or not must be left up to you, not some far off paper pusher who doesn't even know you, let alone examined you, taken your history, and tried to understand you as an individual with a unique set of wants and needs.

Breathing

Breathing can cause a person to have difficulty wearing a face mask safely.

Breathing, being so poorly understood in the general population, it is my suggestion that you not mention breathing at a compliance checkpoint. You may appear perfectly healthy to the untrained eye.

This does not change the fact that shortly after putting on a face mask, you may find yourself in discomfort. It's not worth it.

"I am unable to wear a face mask safely," will get the job done. No need to mention any more at a check-point if this describes your exemption.

The choice to be masked or not must be left up to you, not some far off paper pusher who doesn't

even know you, let alone examined you, taken your history, and tried to understand you as an individual with a unique set of wants and needs.

This Is Not An Exhaustive List Of Conditions

You do not know how my body feels when I put on a face mask. I do not know how your body feels. The best either of us can do is take the other at face value.

There might be a time where your mind is able to be read by another. That time has not arrived.

At present, the sentence *"I am unable to wear a face mask safely,"* must be taken at face value and be a proper foundation for requesting a face mask exemption.

Some conditions may not even be diagnosed yet. You don't know why you really can't tolerate wearing a face mask. That is a matter for you and a trusted practitioner to sort out. It is not a matter for you and me to sort out, nor for you and the person staffing the face mask compliance checkpoint to sort out.

Advanced Applications
Of The Lesson

The Fear Mask And
The "I Surrender" Pose

In *The Apology*, Plato reports the following from Socrates, describing his role as a gadfly as the authorities of Athens sought to put the great teacher to death:

> *"For if you put me to death, you will not easily find another, who, to use a rather absurd figure, attaches himself to the city as a gadfly to a horse, which, though large and well bred, is sluggish on account of his size and needs to be aroused by stinging. I think the god fastened me upon the city in some such capacity, and I go about arousing..."* [102]

A gadfly friend of mine has never done the pose of submission to the great state, the "I surrender" pose.

You know the one where you stick your hands up in the air when someone points a gun at you, exposing your vulnerable torso and midsection.

You know, that "I surrender" pose — the pose that is drilled into you every time you pass through airport security. You must enter the naked body scanner and do the pose of submission. If you don't, you will be barked at, eye-rolled at, and huffed at until you do.

Notably, this "I surrender" pose is merely security theater. It looks like it works. It doesn't actually work. That pose is ineffective security theatre, right alongside the dehumanizing: take off your shoes, get groped, and throw away whatever items you recently bought that happen to be more than the randomly selected 3.3 ounces.

3.4 ounces will take down a plane we are assured. 3.3 ounces can't.

Oh really?

Yes, that's why it must be confiscated. Otherwise, we would never do such an awful thing like confiscate your private property. A half-full 3.4-ounce container can take down a plane too.

Oh really?

Yes, that's why that too must be confiscated. It's for your own safety.

It's fascinating fiction, this US security theater that doesn't actually work. But what it does work at is taking some of the most affluent members of society — air travelers — and bossing them around until they submit. The more affluent you are (to a degree) the more you travel by commercial air. The more you travel by commercial air, the more you get put through the compliance tester and obedience enforcer. This is a predictable way to make the most affluent in a society more compliant.

What a toxic thing for the American experiment and the concept of individual freedom.

You can almost imagine a table of Bush era stooges saying to themselves over beers "What's the stupidest thing we can get people to do?"

"I know. Hold their hands up in the air for no reason like someone is pointing a gun at them."

"Let a stranger go through their underwear."

"No, I've got one better: Let a stranger CONFISCATE their underwear."

"This is way better: Let a stranger take photos of them naked."

"No. Even better. Let a stranger touch them in between the legs."

"No, this is way worse. Get a rattled mother to voluntarily throw away pumped breast milk, because it's a risk to national security, even if that means her baby goes hungry on a flight and screams for three hours."

You now know the "I surrender" pose I mean, right?

Not once has the gadfly done it, despite being a regular traveler by commercial air.

It says a lot about him that he learned about the TSA-implemented pose in the early 2000s and told himself that government would never convince him to do it. He drew a firm line in the sand. A boundary impenetrable.

He would never do the "I surrender" pose for anyone working for the US government, no matter how good of a reason they seemed to be offering him.

That's all there was to it.

You know what else he's never done?

Donned a fear mask.

You know, a fear mask — the pieces of fabric that people have started wearing in response to the top-down national fear mask campaign announced on April 3, 2020.[103]

It's been a popular campaign. Near me, few people were wearing face masks on April 2nd. By the afternoon of April 3, it was hard to find anyone without one.[104-109]

Now, I don't mean to say the gadfly hasn't ever worn a scarf over his face, or a respirator, or a face mask. The guy is as handy as MacGyver, so of course he's worn all that and more. Today he's soldering e-bike parts, to-morrow he's in the middle of the desert keeping his face protected from a dust storm.

But those devices are only really fear masks when you politicize them, when you put a mask on in response to whatever nonsense the CDC, *Fox News*, and *The New York Times* try to provoke in you, when you run from a seasonal virus. You know the one — corona. Then it be-comes a fear mask.

There's a thing about masked faces. They freak people out. People like seeing the full, healthy, relaxed faces of those around them. Reading faces is one way our primal selves avoid danger. Masked faces increase cortisol. They tell you something is wrong. There are several reasons doctors try to avoid masks during hospital rounds, among the reasons: a face is more comforting to a patient.

An additional detail about face masks that is hard to repeat too frequently in this screwy era is that they don't work.

Along with the face mask, has come another fear-induced intervention: the lockdown. The lockdown doesn't appear to work for any respiratory virus. The lockdown certainly doesn't work for Covid-19, which is largely spread in households, not community settings.

Psy Ops (alternately PSYOPS, Psychological Operations, or Psychological Warfare) is a behavior intended to psychologically weaken a target. The US government is renowned for this.

While I don't know what is an intentional Psy Op in my life and what isn't, I know fear is psychologically harmful to me and to those around me. To live in a constant state of fear is hell. It shortens life and reduces the quality of the short life you have.

"When stress is prolonged," writes Aphrodite Matsakis, "The adrenal glands and some of these helping biochemicals can become depleted. This depletion can lead to depression, panic attacks, mood swings, rage reactions, and problems responding appropriately to others."[110]

Notably, the most poignant changes after 9/11 were the ones that worked least, yet created the greatest, most contorted, obeisant behavior in order for a person to travel: the "I surrender" pose and their brethren.

Notably, the most poignant changes after the Ides of March 2020, were the ones that worked least, yet created the greatest, most contorted, obeisant behavior in order for a person to live life: the fear mask and their brethren.

Rooted in fear in order to obtain compliance, these diktats from government do us harm.

Keeping this in mind, it's almost natural for a free person to presume, that in time of crisis, awful advice will come from established government officials talking about best practices, or establishment physicians sharing the standard of care, or the received wisdom of the establishment media telling you what is good for you.

In contrast, the gadfly stings with truth. The work of the gadfly is some of the noblest work that can be done in a society, for it brings others into a more accurate relationship with reality and helps them to live a life that is more effective, more in touch, aware.

That is not readily appreciated by all.

Bloated, with inaction, expert committees, legal liability, risk mitigation, the corpulent hind quarters of the ass barely responds to the gadfly's goading toward the truth. It seeks to pass the rest of life in slumber, to paraphrase Socrates.

The best gadfly is the one who is determined to live life honoring his own boundaries, and to be as truthful as possible with others about where those boundaries are. That person is a natural gadfly. He does not exist to sting another. His mere living of his life, however, is an affront to those who refuse to respect their own boundaries and honestly state those boundaries to others.

It can be no surprise that those who abhor truth, who contort their minds to avoid reality, who want to be coddled in the myth of riskless existence, are those most bothered by the very existence of the gadfly.

Some part of them wants to kill him.

They are "triggered" by him. They build "triggering" into an axiomatic evil, and build morality around the inability to trigger, around the inability to be a gadfly.

Here, coddled society comes into conflict with the free man.

They raise moral arguments against his very nature, against his very existence, to defend themselves from the reminder that they have betrayed their own existence, they have let others repeatedly traverse their own boundaries, they have trampled those boundaries into things unrecognizable.

And yes, in such desperation, they find it a lot easier to blame the gadfly, who they may have never seen their entire lives, but in whose presence they feel twinges of pain, in a way they do not in coddled society.

Irrationally, with great feeling, he must be to blame for the pain. He must be destroyed.

Otherwise, his existence is just too triggering to be moral, in our age that abhors both pain and struggle, almost as much as it abhors truth.

He must be brought to his knees. He must wear the fear mask. He must assume the "I surrender" pose. He must be made to drink the hemlock. He must be killed.

My friend. The Gadfly Majestic.

The Story They Want You To Believe: Why Didn't More Americans Resist?

A brilliant reader points out about American cowardice circa 1913:

> "That idiot Wilson gave us: an unnecessary war, which killed over 100,000 young Americans; the income theft tax; the bank robbers known as the Fed; the League of Nations[111] which morphed into global crooks known as the UN[112]…The sad part is that there was no push back. People accepted the theft then and now. We have been tax slaves for 107 years. Now we are becoming propaganda-virus slaves."

So well put.

Another writes about the confiscation of gold by the US government from the 1930s until the 1970s:

> "I wonder if it was 'prosperity' that made them obedient. But that prosperity was gone during the Great Depression and still people didn't really react to Executive Order 6102."[113]

These two observations share something in common: that people didn't react.

The Grand Lie Of Unanimity

The reaction was massive, but the victor gets to write the history, and that's what the victor wants you to believe: that people didn't react.

That's the best one can do in terms of moral high ground in a democracy: everyone unanimously loved the idea and went along with it. That's the foundation of unanimous consent and voice votes in parliamentary procedure: to pretend division does not exist. It is the method by which thought is silenced and the propagandistic notion of unanimity is forced. Unanimity doesn't exist, except in the most carefully selected grouping of people. Unanimity is a grand lie.

When you are hearing someone referencing unanimity, you can be pretty certain you are speaking to either a liar or a person who hasn't thought through this powerful method of manipulation.

The neo-con wants you to believe everyone supported World War I. The globalist wants you to believe everyone supported the League of Nations and the UN. Virtually the entire economic and financial profession would have you believe everyone supported the formation of the Federal Reserve Bank.[114]

Like Unanimity, "Consensus" Is A Red Flag To The Thinking Man

The word "consensus" accompanied by the word "science," always seems to indicate a person is speaking to the most unsavory of people. There is no grand list of all scientists in the world that would even allow someone to claim that a certain percentage of scientists agree on a given opinion. All claims of unanimity or consensus are dead on arrival to the thinking man, a sign that the speaker can't possibly be serious. Such claims nonetheless are all around us and are too often allowed to go unquestioned.

The Story Of Resistance Written In Family Heirlooms

Executive Order 6102 was used as the legal basis for confiscating gold from Americans. You need only ask someone who was around then, if their family owned any coins during the Great Depression, in order to hear how many "told" Roosevelt to sit on an egg and held onto their gold.

In reality, no one "told" a president anything. It was all done quietly. They might not ever put it in such politicized terms, neither to themselves nor others. They might not say anything pro-Roosevelt or anti-Roosevelt related to gold.

However, anecdote tells the story of many of Americans that refused to turn over their gold. This is among the greatest rebukes possible of that president and his policies. It is an individual stating clearly that they do not trust Roosevelt and his "brain trust" to watch out for their individual needs.

Some families have those contraband coins to this day.

Few grandchildren of the gold hoarders are able to square their unexamined love for the popularly lauded Roosevelt alongside the unexamined disobedience of a grandfather having so much contempt for government, press, and experts. Grandpa had so much contempt that he held onto at least some of his gold. The questions required to square that never get asked. It's a joy to be the one to ask the question that squares that though, and to watch the person in front of your eyes realize the criminality and level of distrust of authority that dear old grandpa exhibited in holding onto the family heirlooms during the depression.

He put the family's long-term financial security ahead of the threat of jail and ahead of the false moralizing of the day.

No, they really don't want those questions to be asked, so they really leave the topic alone. It's far better if everyone just imagines that no era had any conflict except for the present era.

Censoring The Past

All relics telling any other story must be torn down, melted down, and recast down into a lower and less complete version of history that better serves the contemporary status quo.

So much work goes into ignoring the fact that so few people believed the official narrative in the United

States in the 1860s. So few believed the official narrative that hundreds of thousands died. So much work today goes into the narratives "Lincoln is a saint" and "Confederates were racists." To think anything more complex than that makes you a racist. Heaven help those who don't just hold a more sophisticated view of the topic, but know enough to be able to contradict the narrative.

That's what they want you to believe. That's what they need you to believe. Sometimes history repeats itself. Sometimes it "rhymes." They need you to believe a deceitful narrative so that you can't notice the rhymes, so that you continue to believe everything is fine, so that you continue to support the greatest oppression.

Why Is So Much Effort Put Into The Censoring Of History?

Often, the more work that goes into the perpetuation of a total lie, the more important that lie is to have people believe. That Americans didn't resist at any moment in time is a massive lie constantly perpetuated on all manner of topics. Everyone thought everything was okay. It's the fallacy of unanimity.

There's never been a day since 1776 where thirty Americans randomly chosen had a uniform view on any subject. That's the truth. Every moment in human history has been met with resistance. Don't let them tell you any differently.

Identify your boundaries. Communicate your boundaries to others. Defend your boundaries. That is the role of the honest individual in society.

Stick true to your principles and you don't need to worry about whether history rhymes or repeats. You can see how clearly your principles are being violated at such moments.

Tricks Used To Silence True Stories

Beware of every fact, tonality, or scope of debate framed on the airwaves.

Facts — So many know the facts are a lie. So many know experts don't care about data, except data that are useful to manipulate public opinion.

Scope — So many know the frame of debate is an artificial way of manipulating the debate, to convince an onlooker that the onlooker's own truth must be extreme as Beltway Insider One and Beltway Insider Two debate total frivolity and irrelevant nonsense with such great passion that anyone watching is brought to conclude that the topic must really matter. That media trick is a well-known one. So seldom though is the tonality of it all looked at.

Tonality — Even in the very tones the expertly trained mouthpieces use, is a desire to manipulate your views, a desire to manipulate your own tone. Tone has a way of spreading like a social contagion. Tone is the supreme method of manipulation in this finely constructed mechanism of propaganda.

A great machine exists to break your spirit, to get you to deny your values, to get you to let others traverse your boundaries, and for you to sit idly by saying that everything must be okay.

It's not okay.

Protect You Boundaries, Stick To Your Core Values, And All Will Be Okay

Stick true to your core philosophies, let them inform your behavior and it will be okay. Do otherwise and it promises not to be. You will have neither the pride of standing for what you believe nor the joy of coming out of that good fight a victor.

There are millions like you resisting this very moment. There always has been resistance, on every single issue through recorded history. There are tens of millions like you that know how wrong the prevailing narratives of this moment are. The remnant is strong. It is alive and well. It will make it through this moment. And who knows, it might even come to shape this moment.

That isn't the narrative they need you to believe, but it is the truth.

This moment calls on you to look as truthfully as possible at reality and to marshal your resources in support of your deepest beliefs.

A Story That Will Stoke The Courage In You

This is an amazing email sent in by a reader. It is his response to the idea that no one opposed the gold confiscation and bank holidays of Franklin Roosevelt. Be careful. It may stoke the courage in you!

Dear Mr. Stevo,

In 1933, when Roosevelt closed the banks, my great-grandfather, Marion Hezekiah (Kye) Holden, old man Hendricks and old man Chitwood (that's all I ever heard them called) saddled their horses and rode into town ... Atoka, Oklahoma. When they arrived at the bank, they pinwheeled the horses up to the front door. Each man had a Winchester laying across the saddle horn.

There was a US Marshal on either side of the door. Old man Hendricks got down and went into the bank and withdrew all his deposits in gold and silver coin. He returned and remounted. Then Kye did likewise, followed by Chitwood. They were the only ones that got their gold and silver deposits out of the bank.

The US Marshals never moved.

Be blessed.

– H.S., Atoka, Oklahoma

Sticking Up For Others
& Protecting Liberty:
The Niemollerian Buffer

Dear Mr. Stevo,

I would be the exception to what most people do. I read the order and I've printed it out many times, along with supporting documents, for others to read and understand.

I do not own a mask. I've only been challenged a few times. Never once has this resulted in banishment or a loss in services.

As you can see the local "rule," has exemptions. Wearing a mask makes it difficult to breathe, so I demonstrate my opposition openly, and cite the exemption, if challenged by an employee who feels compelled to suffocate slowly.

In the bigger picture, the rules themselves are absurd. I've advised my state representative, health department, and governor that they are way out of bounds. I send videos and articles to the corporations who run the grocery stores, asking them to please stop torturing their employees and warning that ultimately this will adversely affect their bottom line.

Am I on solid ground, or dreaming?

– Winston Smith

"The road to our present hell was paved on 9/11."

German Pastor Martin Niemoller is still remembered for his observation on the world as seen from his vantage point in Germany pre-WW2.

"First they came for the Communists
And I did not speak out
Because I was not a Communist

Then they came for the Socialists
And I did not speak out
Because I was not a Socialist

Then they came for the trade unionists
And I did not speak out
Because I was not a trade unionist

Then they came for the Jews
And I did not speak out
Because I was not a Jew

Then they came for me
And there was no one left
To speak out for me"[115]

Niemoller here describes a Balkanization of society that leads to the diminished view of other humans as less than fully human.

Today, in the United States, as little pockets of political violence erupt and people are murdered for their politics, the consequences of seeing other people as less than fully human are starting to emerge. There is no longer any common morality in the United States. Consequently, anyone can present any awful idea as morality.

It has been observed.

> "When men choose not to believe in God, they do not thereafter believe in nothing, they then become capable of believing in anything."[116]

One such example is the idea that if someone thinks a member of Congress should vote "No" on an issue and you think they should vote "Yes," it is now widely considered inappropriate for you to say "It's just a silly vote that means little in the grand scheme. If I care so much, next time I'll work harder to get my voice heard." It is instead considered appropriate for you to say:

> "Those who disagree with me deserve no rights to speak, no rights to make money, no rights to leave the home unmasked, because they are literally evil, literally racist, literally Satan, literally bigoted, literally Hitler."

Woah!

Watch out snowflake. Those meds might be getting to you. Have you considered asking Dr. Freud to help you taper that dose?

Winston Smith, thank you so much for writing. Your commentary is the exact opposite of what Niemoller describes. It is the opposite of Balkanization. It is the opposite of the trends taking place in the United States today.

Winston Smith, it appears, doesn't just go into a store and shop maskless. He goes into a store, shops maskless, and then chides the managers for not allowing the employees to be maskless. He demands more for his fellow humans.

Winston Smith is the anti-Karen.

He stands up for others. In doing so, he also creates a Niemollerian buffer around himself. In doing so, he defends his own freedom by advancing freedom for another.

A park ranger that I know doesn't seem to care for face masks or the lockdown, but in his "just-doing-my-job" kind of way, the ranger will occasionally bug people. He bugs people about the lockdown orders, because he gets instructed to bug people about the lockdown orders. He gets instructed, because his boss is getting a dozen phone calls a day, from every Karen in town who is troubled by someone having too much fun at the park.

Do you know who never calls him to complain? The people who want to have fun at the park. Those guys wouldn't even dream of it. They just go and have fun elsewhere, if the law comes around looking for trouble.

And this is the way that society, in Fabian fashion, undergoes a long march toward something a lot less wonderful.

How many little guy-lines can the controlling and diminutive Lilliputians string over Gulliver[117] before he notices? How many guy-lines can the Lilliputians string over Gulliver before he has a hard time moving? How many little guy-lines can the Lilliputians string over Gulliver before he can't move at all?

Winston Smith isn't waiting around to find out. He's not only ripping off his guy-lines, he's ripping off the guy-lines of the twenty people around him, whether they like it or not, by giving their Lilliputian boss a piece of his mind.

Thank you, Winston Smith.

You have moved the goal posts and done it in a most wonderful way.

This Is A Book About Self-Esteem

If you know what you want and demand from your life, and you accept those standards, and you know that those are your standards, then there is no one who can deny you those standards but yourself.

That is all there is to it.

Only by backing down, do you not achieve the standards you have for your life.

This is not a book about face masks. This is a book that asks: *Do you love yourself enough to provide yourself with the standard you've set for yourself?*

When it comes to face masks, many want to deny you that standard.

They have all kinds of preconceived notions they have been fed about why it's righteous for them to deny you your sought-after standards.

Well, that's a mere face off of wills. Will you exceed your standards or will you be someone who gets pulled down by a petty tyrant?

You set the stage for the course of your entire life by how you answer that question.

Not how you answer it verbally or on paper, but how you answer it through your actions.

Only for the overly literal is it really a book about face masks. Face mask policies are a gift from the year 2020 that allow a person to challenge their self-esteem and rise to the occasion.

2020 promises to be the most formative year of this century to date, in the cause of freedom, for it is the year that has demanded the most of free individuals.

I anticipate that I will cherish my personal advancements from this year for many years to come and I anticipate that every free man walking the earth will feel the same way about this crucible of a year.

The Ritual Cleansing
Of Mask Burning

Burning Man has an oral tradition that circulates among the returning burners with a penchant for stories.

One night a man sat in his apartment with a few friends, having a drink and bemoaned the woman who had left him. He was advised to get over her.

How could he get over her with all her stuff still here in his apartment?

He started pointing around the room at all her things. That piece of garbage in the corner, that thing hanging from the wall, all that stuff in the bathroom crowding out every little shelf. She's never come to pick it up no matter how many times he's asked her. She's moved on.

Well, someone chimed in, "Why not just take it all down to the beach right now and burn it all?"

A few drinks later that's what they did.

And on the year anniversary of that bonfire of the vanities, the others in the room that night took their ex's stuff down to the same San Francisco beach and burned it.

This is how Burning Man began.

How cathartic of an experience to watch the symbols of a despicable era of the past consumed by fire and to never be with you again.

What a clean break and with a little excitement as well.

On the night of Oct 7, 2020, a group of orthodox Jews in Borough Park, Brooklyn gathered as a community and burned their face masks.[118-120]

What's stopping you from doing the same?

Do you fear the catharsis that would bring?

Do you fear the clean break from the past?

Why Technocrats Believe In Face Masks

"My name is Ozymandias, King of Kings;

Look on my Works, ye Mighty, and despair!"

– Percy Shelley [121]

There's a group of people who walk the earth who don't just believe that life can be improved by humans, they take it a step further.

They believe humans can be improved.

While this sentence may not seem irksome to you, because it is so commonplace, I hope in a few paragraphs you'll see how truly twisted it is.

Most people who observe nature and humanity — the overwhelming majority of people walking the planet — learn some version of "If it ain't broke, then don't try to fix it." Many religions teach this.

Man is created in the image of God, but is fallen.

Man has perfection in him if he can find it.

All creation is of the Creator.

There can be a religious aspect to it, but there are also people who will have no religious reason for an "If it ain't broke, then don't try to fix it" view of man and nature.

A conservative might not like new government regulation when a private contract between two people works just fine in almost all scenarios.

A hippie might not see a doctor for 30 years because he doesn't have a health problem and can't imagine the benefit of exposing himself to big pharma's salesman in his community, the local doctor.

A farmer might do the same, to the point where their politics may not converge, but their "If it ain't broke, don't try to fix it" sensibilities overlap perfectly.

An inner-city grandma might feel the exact same way.

An immigrant grandpa may as well.

The sensibility to just leave things alone and the humbleness required to say "It's not perfect, but its good enough" is pervasive throughout American society and globally.

Then there are a different group of people.

That is the 5%, 10%, maybe even 20% who comprise the technocratic class and who either never learn that humbleness or learned to do away with that same sense of humbleness.

In that humbleness, "If it ain't broke don't try to fix it," is a connectedness to reality that can seldom be spoken of by a technocrat, because they don't really understand it.

If you mess with something that works, there's a good chance you won't be able to get it back to normal again.

That is true in many areas of life. The mechanic rarely gets your car as good as new. When he starts to play with one thing, something else starts to go, or he pre-emptively points out another thing that has lasted 8 years just fine, but is soon "about to go."

Similarly, no matter what they say, the doctor never gets your hips as good as new, and heck, his bionic knee implants might feel better than the old arthritic things you knew, but their functionality is no comparison to the real thing.

Not until the doctor takes his own medicine and gets his own knees done will he come to understand what you mean when you say your knees aren't as good as new. You might even be a little sore about it because that's not the outcome you were told to be able to expect.

No, the technocrat makes a living out of ignoring reality and pretending that humbleness is a quaint term that does not apply to someone as well-intentioned and well-trained as him.

And there is the rub.

That is where idealism and reality conflict.

Yes, of course, the technocrat can mean well, but good intentions don't go very far in reality.

Before setting into motion the harsh realities of cause and effect that are reality and life, nature doesn't hit the pause button and ask "Did you mean to do that?"

No, to the contrary, causes have effects, actions have consequences, and it is you that set those in motion.

Often, "I didn't mean to," will mean little in a situation where you should have known better.

The technocrat is he who should know better and instead resolves, to go through life suggesting implicitly and explicitly that outcomes are irrelevant and intentions are fundamental.

That's some pretty serious Lala Land that a double-digit percentage of the Western population seeks to live in through their thoughts and actions.

And it is a largely Western concept: this professionalization of all and this rule by a technocratic class.

How divorced from reality it is. How refreshing reality can be when one is drowning in the mire of such cluelessness run amuck, as the idea that intentions matter and outcomes do not, which has so taken our culture by storm.

In the "If it ain't broke, then don't try to fix it," sensibility of the world, it is before you try and fix something that your intentions still matter.

It is in the bedroom that you decide whether or not you want a baby.

It is in the courtship that you decide what kind of life you want ahead for you.

It is in the decision to snooze two more hours or rise, to make the bed or to leave it unkempt, to be diligent with your life or to be neglectful, that you demonstrate your intentions.

After you mess up grandma's television set, grandma's car, or grandma's knees, is not the time to say "oops" and talk about intentions.

That's how a weasel behaves and a forthright and decent person knows that intimately, which is why technocrats don't get a lot of respect outside of the technocratic circles they travel in.

How many times have we all heard a technocrat explain that he is just — misunderstood?

Many. We just don't realize it all that often, in the midst of their sophisticated ways of saying so.

Truth is, they aren't misunderstood. Plenty of salt-of-the-earth people know perfectly well what a technocrat means to do. He means to ignore the wise "If it ain't broken, then don't try to fix it," and then when his fix goes awry, he means to escape culpability by speaking about his intentions, and preparing everyone to trust his next fix, which he assures everyone is sure to work this time around.

If it were left at that, that might be acceptable, but it rarely is these days.

Rarely do technocrats let their ideas get challenged in the marketplace of ideas, to get evaluated, and then adopted by individuals freely or alternately ignored and perhaps derided by individuals freely.

No, many technocrats have no such sense of decency. Instead of trying to win in the marketplace of ideas, the territory of the free man and one of the joys of a free society, they figure out how to get a man with a badge and a gun involved.

Once that happens, even among the few generous people willing to give a technocrat a chance, all presumption of good intent must be done away with.

If their argument is so great, why would anyone need a billion dollar marketing budget and a half billion worth of armed and trained quasi-military civilian government commandos to get you to hear their good ideas?

That's where we are in the year 2020.

Your wonderful immune system. Your wonderful body. Your wonderful ability to inhale and exhale. That can all be improved upon with a 10-cent polypropylene mask from Wuhan province. That's what the technocrats assure us.

It is another example of lacking humility and the contact with reality provided by "If it ain't broke, then don't try to fix it." Then there is the added idea that there is an even better way for the technocrat to improve life, even better than the "mandatory" face masks: just put every-one's life on hold in mandatory lockdowns.

You salt-of-the-earth people weren't doing anything all that special with your life anyway, were you?

Yes, in 2020, we all saw how sociopathic the technocrats got and saw it pretty quickly as they implemented "lockdowns for thee, but not for me," and turned that crank tighter and tighter.

Why do technocrats advocate so ardently for face masks?

Because they know no humbleness and because they don't comprehend the common decency of "If it ain't broke, then don't try to fix it."

Conclusion

If The Vaccine Comes And You Are Still Wearing A Face Mask, You're In For A World Of Pain

If I were to lay in bed for the next twenty years, and to then rise, I would not have much strength in my muscles to do the activities I once enjoyed.

I might collapse onto the ground, with my poor quivering atrophied muscles shocked by the sudden immense force that they have been called on to exert in this untrained state.

If I trained every day for a week, I might be able to get out of bed again. If I trained every day for a month, I might be able to go for a walk again.

It's going to take some doing to work through that kind of rust, and to train yourself out of that kind of neglect — but if you know that going in, maybe that little bit of effort won't be so bad.

You've done harder things. There was a time in your life, early on, when you spent every waking hour for about six months trying to figure out how to just roll your body over. You were also working on learning other tasks at the same time. Imagine how simple that movement probably is for you today and how hard it once was.

For a year, maybe a year-and-a-half, you tried your best to figure out how to balance head atop neck, atop shoulder, atop spine, atop hips, atop femur, atop knees, atop tibia, atop ankles, atop all those little movements in those cute little feet and toes that it took to keep you balanced that first time you let go and stood, and then dared to take a step. Why'd you do it? Because it felt as natural as walking out into the fresh air and feeling the sunshine on your entire face. Just feels right, this thing we call freedom.

To this day, you still probably trip and fall from time to time. Balance and coordination are a lifelong endeavor. Many efforts are a lifelong endeavor that not only stop growing, but atrophy, and even die if neglected.

Would the most innocent, lump of happiness and love that makes up a child ever sabotage her own growth, her own progress, her own advancement toward being a full, free, and capable part of this world?

I've never heard of that child.

Then what would cause any adult to do that? Somewhere along the way something changes in some people.

It took you about two years to learn how to grasp a thing as simple as a pencil, and another two years of work before you could bring any precision to the process, perhaps even longer. To this day, you probably still have to work pretty hard, if you're going to operate a pencil with much precision.

I'm not asking you to do anything that hard at all, nothing as hard as the work it took you to learn how to operate a pencil, which when you think about it is a pretty amazing accomplishment. Compared to all the thousands of challenges like these, that you've worked so hard at and accomplished, this one is a walk in the proverbial park.

For twenty years, the average and above-average American alike have been laying in bed, ever since those planes hit the World Trade Center and government said "Go to your room. We're in charge now."

It can be no surprise that some muscles have since atrophied. The emergency they said they were handling never came to an end. The terror alerts never stopped. Some people never stopped talking about them. To this day, I don't know what those terror alerts mean or why they matter, and not for the life of me do I care.

People have tried to explain it to me, perhaps not realizing that I stopped listening to them about twenty seconds before they started explaining, right around the moment where their tonality shifted away from the "I-am-telling-you-something-sincere-or-original" voice to the "I-am-now-delivering-a-preprogrammed-message" voice.

We still have alerts. We still have security at airports that touch passengers' private parts "for the safety of all." We still have a two decade unending war. We still have an even bigger military with all its parasitic appendages that a United States President and General once called the "military industrial complex" in his nationally televised farewell address on January 17, 1961.[122]

He, Dwight Eisenhower, knew that topic better than anyone and appealed to the American public on national television about it, yet today it is a conversational topic relegated to those pejoratively deemed "oddballs," which is exactly how some special interest groups would like it to be.

Because of the failures of many, a generation ago, in their own lives that allowed security theater to be commonplace in America, all the leftover nonsense of the last twenty years are problems that remain today as temporal and qualitative taxations on daily life. But some people do not comply. Some refuse to lift their hands in the "I surrender" pose.

They have not been laying in bed twenty years. Their muscles are strong. They have not neglected to fight the fight that so many others ran from. Consequently, these people who stood up twenty years ago and continue to do so to this day, have felt little of the tyranny that is American security theater.

People like that saw the goofy face mask order on the horizon and laughed:

> "You think I'm scared of an unenforced face mask order? I stared down low paid, poorly trained, uninformed, uniformed TSA government thugs from 2002 to 2020 who were told that they were the front line in the War on Ter-

ror and that I must be a baby killing terrorist if I didn't comply with their every word. And I did that during 40 trips each year, both ways. You think I'm scared of this face mask hype?"

People like that aren't scared. They've been building their muscles. They've seen some of the worst this country has offered its citizens over the last two decades and have survived uncowed and unscathed.

What happened to everyone else?

You may have been one of those who stayed in bed. Perhaps you are ready to start working those muscles again.

"If you're like me, you want your heroes full-throated and unflinching," writes the full-throated and unflinching Becky Akers.

I don't expect to ever see her in a fear mask. I don't expect to ever see her lining up for a Bill Gates approved anti-viral regimen. I don't expect to ever see her complying with the government's "mandatory" recommendations.

Some days, dozens of people write me to tell me their stories from the corona compliance checkpoint. Boy does that give me inspiration. It inspires me not because they aren't wearing face masks, it inspires me because I know they are 1.) identifying their boundaries, 2.) communicating their boundaries, and 3.) defending their boundaries.

That is an applicable skill in the face of any request from government, from an employer, from a customer, from a spouse, from a thief, from a parent, from a child, from a friend, from anyone.

It's not just about government. Government is not to blame, but you might be.

It's about being honest with yourself and with others as you live your life. There is no freedom any other way. Even though they may not be stated the exact same way, all attempts at freedom succeed because they focus on this principle of identifying, communicating, and defending personal boundaries.

I'm happy when I hear these stories because these stories are bigger than masks. These stories are about people building their most valuable muscles in ensuring their individual freedom.

Yeah, I get it, it's also about masks and exemptions and valid reasons to be able to stop hiding in your house, and why you shouldn't be scared to exercise your valid exemptions.

The millions of Americans with valid exemptions get to rise up, each morning, thankful for the condition that they may have once felt was a disability, because in this moment they are able to advance and defend human freedom in their own lives in a way that so many others are afraid to do without the law on their side, and it's about so much more too.

Because in that process, you really have a chance to bulk up those muscles.

I pity the fool who isn't taking that chance.

I don't know what the future holds. No one does. But some of those necromancers, charlatans, and algorithm buggers claim to have a crystal ball telling them their future. They are saying pretty clearly what their plan for your future as well.

It's a scary future they describe.

I know quite a few people who won't take part in that future, because they've trained every chance they could, every day they could, for many years of their lives. I know others, many others, who are new to all this, but who won't take part in that future because they have been training every day that they can, every opportunity they can, since the first time someone told them to wear a fear mask. Some may have even had their change of heart this very moment.

They laughed: "You want me to do what?"

And then they never did that thing that was so foolish an idea that they laughed out loud at it.

That's real life training — perhaps the most vital training — doing what you want, and not doing what you don't want to do. It's honest. The deepest honesty may exist in disobedience. The two are not antonyms, no matter what virtually every authority figure in human history would have you believe.

Those who walk through every retail door they want as a paying customer, and every church door they want as a parishioner, and every space they want as a visitor, and figure out how to do it without the mask — even if they only start demanding that standard for themselves starting this moment — those are the ones who won't take a vaccine. Those are the ones who will know their boundaries, know how to communicate their boundaries, know how to defend their boundaries, and consequently, will be ready for whatever comes next.

They aren't saying to themselves "I'll lay in bed six more months, and if it's really bad then, I'll stand up for the first time in twenty years." Some people, unfortunately, are telling themselves that exact fairy tale as they press the snooze button and roll over, getting comfortable with everything happening around them.

I don't know what comes next.

You don't know what comes next.

But I know the tools I need to be a free man in this world.

And do I ever feel lucky to be able to train with them so much this year.

A pope once wrote "Let us thank God that He makes us live among the present problems. It is no longer permitted to anyone to be mediocre."

I like that.

Who's with me?

Afterword

If You Announce Your VIP Status To The World, The World Will Accommodate Your VIP Status

Recently at a hardware store that I called ahead of time, asking for recognition of a face mask exemption, the manager notified all employees that a customer would be coming in unmasked.

I did so, true to my word.

When an employee then got after me about the face masks, he was quickly reprimanded by that same manager and not once but twice sought me out and offered sincere and lengthy apologies for giving me a hard time.

As part of my political consulting work, I have advanced presidential candidates, senators, and congressmen. I go ahead of them and make sure all appropriate accommodations are in place and that they receive frictionless, white glove treatment in all of the usual spots where regular people encounter friction.

It has always amazed me how willing people are to make accommodation when simply asked. Just asking really goes a long way.

My suggestion to you is to do what a VIP would do, and just let others know what you want. You don't need to be a VIP in order to tell others what you want. You just need to be someone dedicated to communicating honestly to another.

You could also do what handicapped people have long done: stating what you want to a person in a position to provide you with what you want. That responsibility has been drilled into the minds of handicap people: if they do not ask for accommodation, there is no possible way that a person who does not live their life would ever know what kind of accommodation they would need.

To pretend that another person can read your mind is utter nonsense and handicapped people for time immemorial have had this burden of honest communication to bear. It is enshrined into law as well that it is appropriate to make certain accommodations for the handicapped. It is debatable how much federal laws such as the *Americans with Disabilities Act* serve the interest of individuals with disabilities, but something it is likely to achieve is to force the topic of individual accommodations into the training of virtually every customer-facing employee in the United States at any company of a certain size.

Just like you don't have to be a VIP in order to tell others what you want, you also don't have to be handicapped in order to tell others what you want. Quite to the contrary, anyone can communicate the level of directness and honesty that VIPs and the handicapped have both been expected to demonstrate if they were to have their needs and wants met.

That is what honest people have long done — people committed to being honest to themselves and honest to others as well — simply telling others what they want.

The Bible speaks to this courage to utilize this honesty and the rich rewards that such courage and honesty provide. In Matthew 7:7 we find the well-known observation about how life works "Ask, and it shall be given you; seek, and ye shall find; knock, and it shall be opened unto you."

Sometimes all you have to do is knock on a door to be let through that door.

At the heart of this method is honesty. It is 1.) honestly identifying your own boundaries, 2.) honestly communicating your own boundaries, and 3.) honestly defending your own boundaries.

That is some of the most important honesty that can take place, and an honesty that is often lacking in our contemporary era where we are so often told it is "rude" or "selfish" to tell another person what you want. It is neither. It is honest.

Correspondingly, it is neither rude nor selfish for another person to tell you "No," in response to your request. They have the right to tell you that they don't want to comply with your request.

Rather than honesty, what daily life is often full of is passive-aggression.

"Passive-aggressive" is a word thrown around in popular culture, to the point where it's meaning is approximately: that which I do not like.

It's meaning is far more nuanced and sinister for it is the embodiment in action of deceitful thoughts.

Claudia Zayfert, PhD and Jason C. DeViva, PhD[123] describe passive-aggression in a way that so clearly demonstrates the fundamental deceit underlying it.

> "Passive–aggressive behavior is acting aggressively toward a person in a way that makes it hard for them to see our intentions or blame us for the outcome. Someone who is being passive–aggressive may tell a friend she will do something, never really intending to follow through, and then not do it, coming up with an excuse that leaves her blameless. Passive–aggressive people may think, 'I really want to tell you this, but that would be difficult or uncomfortable, so I'll tell you something else but then do what I wanted to do in the first place.'

> "The attraction of passive–aggressive behavior is that it allows us to meet our needs and ignore the other person's needs without his knowing. The major drawback is that people often figure out that there is something false about either what the passive–aggressive person is saying or what he's doing. One patient described passive–aggressive behavior by a friend as 'smil-

ing while he screwed me.' Not surprisingly, passive–aggressive behavior often is damaging to relationships."

Often, people in customer service roles want to give you exactly what you want. You just need to ask for it clearly, ask for it properly, and ask for it nicely.

Ways to accomplish all three of those are contained in these pages, pages that I hope you've found most insightful and enjoyable.

Appendix

Reminder: The CDC Says Face Masks Don't Stop Covid

The US Center for Disease Control and Prevention (CDC) has an estimated 15,000 in its workforce; some 88 of them work on *Emerging Infectious Diseases*, a highly regarded, peer-reviewed journal of epidemiology,[124] published by the CDC.

April 3, 2020 — CDC Face Mask Order

On April 3, 2020, the CDC announced that everyone should wear face masks, wash their hands, and clean surfaces in order to prevent the spread of Covid-19.[125]

CDC 4/3/20: Wear Masks To Fight Covid

On April 3, 2020, the CDC advised "Everyone should wear a cloth face cover when they have to go out in public, for example to the grocery store or to pick up other necessities." Private and governmental policies across the US and internationally were crafted according to this statement.[126]

CDC 4/3/20: Wash Hands To Fight Covid

On April 3, 2020, the CDC advised "Wash your hands often with soap and water for at least 20 seconds especially after you have been in a public place, or after blowing your nose, coughing, or sneezing."

CDC 4/3/20: Clean Surfaces To Fight Covid

On April 3, 2020, the CDC advised "Clean AND disinfect frequently touched surfaces daily. This includes tables, door-knobs, light switches, countertops, handles, desks, phones, keyboards, toilets, faucets, and sinks."

May 2020 — Researchers Prove The Opposite

May 2020, Dr. Jingyi Xiao, an epidemiologist from the University of Hong Kong, and her colleagues, ran a paper entitled "Nonpharmaceutical Measures for Pandemic Influenza in Nonhealthcare Settings[127]—Personal Protective and Environmental Measures" at *Emerging Infectious Diseases*,[128] in which they sought to separate myth from reality and to demonstrate what data-driven measures can be helpful in preventing the spread of Covid-19. Xiao's research showed the opposite of the April 3, 2020, statements from the CDC to be true.

Superior Methodology

Xiao's efforts began with more diligent and rigorous methodology than recent reviewers who came before:

> "We searched 4 databases (Medline, PubMed, EMBASE, and CENTRAL) for literature in all languages. We aimed to identify randomized controlled trials (RCTs) of each measure for laboratory-confirmed influenza outcomes for each of the measures because RCTs provide the highest quality of evidence."

Throughout 2020, it has been easy for low-quality Covid research to get published and then circulated through the media, entirely out of context. This has been detrimental in a time when high quality and dependable information would be most useful in the protection of life and livelihood in 2020.

Consequently, Xiao does not treat every study the same. Randomized controlled trials with laboratory confirmed outcomes were the standard their review of the literature sought. Rather than cherry-picking the studies with fashionable results, they sought truth and quality over political correctness and assessed the gold standard studies. Not surprisingly, in doing so, Xiao produced the exact opposite results of what you would find from *Fox News*, *The New York Times*, Google, or their many clones.

Xiao unsurprisingly reports what researchers of randomized controlled trials with laboratory-confirmed outcomes have long known:

> "Although mechanistic studies support the potential effect of hand hygiene or face masks, evidence from 14 randomized controlled trials of these measures did not support a substantial effect on transmission of

laboratory-confirmed influenza. We similarly found limited evidence on the effectiveness of improved hygiene and environmental cleaning. We identified several major knowledge gaps requiring further research, most fundamentally an improved characterization of the modes of person-to-person transmission."

You read that right:

1.) It doesn't matter if you sanitize surfaces;

2.) It doesn't matter if you wash your hands;

3.) Masks don't work.

CDC Journal 5/1/20: Sanitizing Surfaces Doesn't Protect Against Covid-19

Sanitizing surfaces is effective for the prevention of gastrointestinal illnesses, but it doesn't protect from Covid:

> "Although we found no evidence that surface and object cleaning could reduce influenza transmission, this measure does have an established impact on prevention of other infectious diseases."

CDC Journal 5/1/20: Washing Your Hands Doesn't Protect Against Covid

Similarly, hand washing is useful for the prevention of gastrointestinal illness, but the laboratory-confirmed, randomized controlled trials show that it is not useful in the prevention of Covid:

> "Hand hygiene is a widely used intervention and has been shown to effectively reduce the transmission of gastrointestinal infections and respiratory infections. However, in our systematic review, updating the findings of Wong et al., we did not find evidence of a major effect of hand hygiene on laboratory-confirmed influenza virus transmission. Nevertheless, hand hy-

giene might be included in influenza pandemic plans as part of general hygiene and infection prevention."

CDC Journal 5/1/20: Masks Don't Work

Face masks might help prevent the spread of some infections, but there's no proof that they work with Covid-19 or influenza:

"We did not find evidence that surgical-type face masks are effective in reducing laboratory-confirmed influenza transmission, either when worn by infected persons (source control) or by persons in the general community to reduce their susceptibility. However, as with hand hygiene, face masks might be able to reduce the transmission of other infections and therefore have value in an influenza pandemic when healthcare resources are stretched."

CDC Journal 5/1/20: Face Masks Don't Work When Worn By The Sick Either

Some say face masks should be worn by the infected, not the healthy. In doing so, they can prevent infected people from transmitting the virus to the healthy. Xiao found no such evidence of this. Rather than relying on datasets based on questionnaires such as "Did you suffer from the sniffles last week?" Xiao, in examining this issue, only looked at laboratory-confirmed cases and found no proof that people sick with Covid or influenza should war masks either:

"There is limited evidence for their effectiveness in preventing influenza virus transmission either when worn by the infected person for source control or when worn by uninfected persons to reduce exposure. Our systematic review found no significant effect of face masks on transmission of laboratory-confirmed influenza."

CDC Journal 5/1/20: Don't Wear A Dirty Mask, It Can INCREASE The Risk Of Covid Transmission

Xiao takes it a step further, saying not only are face masks unhelpful in stopping the spread of Covid-19, they can actually increase the risk of transmission:

> "Proper use of face masks is essential because improper use might increase the risk for transmission. Thus, education on the proper use and disposal of used face masks, including hand hygiene, is also needed."

What Is "Proper Use?"

Xiao cites a World Health Organization (WHO) notice from 2009 entitled "Advice on the use of masks in the community setting in Influenza A (H1N1) outbreaks" that offers some well-established advice for proper mask use. Again Xiao has demonstrated that proper mask use does not stop Covid-19 but to cite the WHO the great risk of the mask is that transmission is increased: "Using a mask incorrectly however, may actually increase the risk of transmission, rather than reduce it."

The following from WHO is listed as behavior that can increase transmission:[129]

- Touching mouth and nose
- Touching a mask in use
- Touching a clean mask with unwashed hands
- Not washing hands every time after touching a dirty mask
- Wearing a mask that is not new and clean
- Continuing to wear a mask after it has become damp, instead of immediately replacing it
- Re-using a single-use mask
- Not discarding a single-use mask immediately upon removal, as opposed to leaving it in the immediate environment

Have you seen even one person follow that protocol in 2020? Proper mask protocol doesn't stop there either. Rather than informing the public that such behaviors may actually help spread Covid, the most vocal instead demand that everyone be masked, regardless of the potential negative impact it may have in increasing the transmission of Covid-19.

CDC Journal 5/1/20: Covering Your Mouth Doesn't Even Seem To Work

Etiquette in many places says you cover your mouth when you sneeze or cough. Xiao went so far as to investigate this also, finding such respiratory etiquette unhelpful in preventing the transmission of Covid, and encouraging others to take up that area of research:

> "Respiratory etiquette is often listed as a preventive measure for respiratory infections. However, there is a lack of scientific evidence to support this measure. Whether respiratory etiquette is an effective non-pharmaceutical intervention in preventing influenza virus transmission remains questionable, and worthy of further research."

Caveat: Xiao Did Not Look At N95 And P2 Respirators

Focusing on the most pressing matters that relate to the greatest number of people, Xiao looked at face masks and not respirators. Respirators come with their own warning. They, too, require their own hygiene and fit protocol in order to be effective, protocol seldom followed, among the general public.

Xiao writes:

> "We did not consider the use of respirators in the community. Respirators are tight-fitting masks that can protect the wearer from fine particles and should provide better protection against influenza virus exposures when properly worn because of higher filtration efficiency. However, respirators, such as N95 and P2 masks, work best when they are fit-tested, and these masks will be in limited supply during the next pandemic."

Who Is More Credible —
Political Hacks Or Gold Standard Scientists?

It would look, on the surface, like the CDC is contradicting itself. One organ of the CDC said one thing in April and another organ said something else in May, which would not be the first confusing message from the CDC. One may feel torn between who to believe. That need not be the case at all.

You have the top brass at the CDC, composed of political hacks saying to wear something, anything, as long as it vaguely resembles a mask. Their statements shift whenever it's expedient to them. Then, in contrast, you have the peer-reviewed scientists pointing to the well-established and long-established fact that masks don't work for reducing coronavirus transmission.

I don't know what the political hacks are trying to pull or why, and I don't particularly need to know in order to understand why not to trust political hacks. What I know is that what they are saying is predictably inaccurate. This is the case for much of what political hacks say. Just because it comes from the hacks does not make it wrong, but hacks have a bad track record when it comes to science. They just don't have a primary penchant for truth. If they did, they would not be political hacks.

Face masks don't work in preventing the spread of Covid. The science on that is well-established.

2020 Has Been A Year Of Superstition, Not Science

Many of the weird, OCD, germophobe, anti-social, hypochondriac maneuvers that have become commonplace in 2020 are rooted in superstition, but not science. While these interventions may be the advice of those reading *Fox News* marquees or *New York Times* headlines, they are not data-driven interventions backed by peer-reviewed, laboratory-confirmed, randomized controlled trials. Those trials say something clearly different.

Face mask orders are the territory of the science-denier, the anti-logician, the mob with torches ready to punish Copernicus for applying the scientific method and thinking according to his findings. It's not me saying that, that's just the 14 gold standard studies used by Xiao et al.

Knowing This, What Will You Do?

Now I have tremendous regard for those who will take this knowledge and evangelize. I also have tremendous praise for those who will take that knowledge and crash the gates. My method has been to encourage people with exemptions to say the words *"I am unable to wear a face mask safely."* Thousands have successfully used this technique. Millions can successfully use it. One free person at a time, these lockdowns come to an end, not when any blue ribbon committee says they end.

Conclusion: The Experts Know A Lot Less Than They Have Led Us To Believe

Xiao provides a useful slice of humble pie to the people who suddenly became Covid experts and tinpot dictators this spring. The aggressive mask-police don't know as much as they think they do. The "experts" that the aggressive mask police are getting their info from don't either.

Unfortunately, this sober appraisal doesn't sell advertising, fund studies, or make careers, so instead of being the most cited study of 2020, Xiao has practically been ignored.

Perhaps in your own circle of friends, you can change this by sharing this Xiao's work and this book.

And while you're at it, please also send me your tales from the face mask compliance checkpoint, and help me put an end to this tyranny.

WHO Says We Are Doing It Wrong

Xiao's study "Nonpharmaceutical Measures for Pandemic Influenza in Nonhealthcare Settings—Personal Protective and Environmental Measures" cites the following World Health Organization guidance, which provides effective protocols for methods of usage that make face masks as effective as possible. These protocols are entirely ignored in the farcical face mask guidances of 2020.

Advice On The Use Of Masks In The Community Setting In Influenza A (H1N1) Outbreaks

Interim Guidance

3 May 2009

This document provides interim guidance on the use of masks in communities that have reported community-level outbreaks caused by the new Influenza A(H1N1) virus. It will be revised as more data become available.

Background

At present, evidence suggests that the main route of human-to-human transmission of the new Influenza A (H1N1) virus is via respiratory droplets, which are expelled by speaking, sneezing or coughing.

Any person who is in close contact (approximately 1 metre) with someone who has influenza-like symptoms (fever, sneezing, coughing, running nose, chills, muscle ache etc) is at risk of being exposed to potentially infective respiratory droplets.

In healthcare settings, studies evaluating measures to reduce the spread of respiratory viruses suggest that the use of masks could reduce the transmission of influenza. Advice on the use of masks in healthcare settings is accompanied by information on additional measures that may have impact on its effectiveness, such as training on correct use, regular supplies and proper disposal facilities. In the community, however, the benefits of wearing masks has not been established, especially

271

in open areas, as opposed to enclosed spaces while in close contact with a person with influenza-like symptoms.

Nonetheless, many individuals may wish to wear masks in the home or community setting, particularly if they are in close contact with a person with influenza-like symptoms, for example while providing care to family members. Furthermore, using a mask can enable an individual with influenza-like symptoms to cover their mouth and nose to help contain respiratory droplets, a measure that is part of cough etiquette.

Using a mask incorrectly however, may actually increase the risk of transmission, rather than reduce it. If masks are to be used, this measure should be combined with other general measures to help prevent the human-to-human transmission of influenza, training on the correct use of masks and consideration of cultural and personal values.

General Advice

It is important to remember that in the community setting the following general measures may be more important than wearing a mask in preventing the spread of influenza.

For individuals who are well:

Maintain distance of at least 1 metre from any individual with influenza-like symptoms, and:

- refrain from touching mouth and nose;
- perform hand hygiene frequently, by washing with soap and water or using an alcohol-based handrub, especially if touching the mouth and nose and surfaces that are potentially contaminated;
- reduce as much as possible the time spent in close contact with people who might be ill;
- reduce as much as possible the time spent in crowded settings;
- improve airflow in your living space by opening windows as much as possible.

For individuals with influenza-like symptoms:

- stay at home if you feel unwell and follow the local public health recommendations;
- keep distance from well individuals as much as possible (at least 1 metre);
- cover your mouth and nose when coughing or sneezing, with tissues or other suitable materials, to contain respiratory secretions. Dispose of the material immediately after use or wash it. Clean hands immediately after contact with respiratory secretions!
- improve airflow in your living space by opening windows as much as possible.

If masks are worn, proper use and disposal is essential to ensure they are potentially effective and to avoid any increase in risk of transmission associated with the incorrect use of masks. The following information on correct use of masks derives from the practices in healthcare settings:

- place mask carefully to cover **mouth and nose** and tie securely to minimise any gaps between the face and the mask
- while in use, avoid touching the mask
  - whenever you touch a used mask, for example when removing or washing, clean hands by washing with soap and water or using an alcohol-based handrub
- replace masks with a new clean, dry mask as soon as they become damp/humid
- do not re-use single-use masks
  - discard single-use masks after each use and dispose of them immediately upon removing.

Although some alternative barriers to standard medical masks are frequently used (e.g. cloth mask, scarf, paper masks, rags tied over the nose and mouth), there is insufficient information available on their effectiveness. If such alternative barriers are used, they should only be used once or, in the case of cloth masks, should be cleaned thoroughly between each use (i.e. wash with normal household detergent at normal temperature). They should be removed immediately after caring for the ill. Hands should be washed immediately after removal of the mask.

Remember What A Wiser Generation Warned Us About Corona Hysterics: The Story Of Chicken Little

There's a tale from my childhood that goes back many generations in European culture and can be traced back long before that, with components of it and lessons akin to it being seen in many cultures around the world.

The story contains some of the most important lessons that a generation can pass down about times of perceived crisis.

The idea of it is that the wise one controls his emotions. The wise one does not counter-rationally let his emotions lead him. The wise one does not follow others who are being led by their emotions. The wise one does not let down their guard in the midst of hysterics. The wise one does not part with all that is precious to them because someone is being emotional. Led by emotion in perceived crisis, you might win a victory or two. Even a broken watch is right twice a day. It never ends well for people who let themselves be led through life in such a way.

It is a warning from the past about exactly the type of historical moment that is upon us.

> Chicken Little likes to walk in the woods. She likes to look at the trees. She likes to smell the flowers. She likes to listen to the birds singing.
>
> One day while she is walking an acorn falls from a tree, and hits the top of her little head.
>
> "My, oh, my, the sky is falling. I must run and tell the lion about it," says Chicken Little and begins to run.
>
> She runs and runs. By and by she meets the hen.
>
> "Where are you going?" asks the hen.

"Oh, Henny Penny, the sky is falling and I am going to the lion to tell him about it."

"How do you know it?" asks Henny Penny.

"It hit me on the head, so I know it must be so," says Chicken Little.

"Let me go with you!" says Henny Penny. "Run, run."

So the two run and run until they meet Ducky Lucky.

"The sky is falling," says Henny Penny. "We are going to the lion to tell him about it.

"How do you know that?" asks Ducky Lucky.

"It hit Chicken Little on the head," says Henny Penny.

"May I come with you?" asks Ducky Lucky.

"Come," says Henny Penny.

So all three of them run on and on until they meet Foxey Loxey.

"Where are you going?" asks Foxey Loxey.

"The sky is falling and we are going to the lion to tell him about it," says Ducky Lucky.

"Do you know where he lives?" asks the fox.

"I don't," says Chicken Little.

"I don't," says Henny Penny.

"I don't," says Ducky Lucky.

"I do," says Foxey Loxey. "Come with me and I can show you the way."

He walks on and on until he comes to his den.

"Come right in," says Foxey Loxey.

They all go in, but they never, never come out again.

A Non-Exhaustive List
Of Legal Resources By State

Below is a collection of organizations that advocate for greater individual liberty. Some of them litigate. All of them can be expected to be in contact with litigators in their state and region.

Approached properly, all are likely to be willing to consider thinking through any legal matter you bring them. In doing so, they may at least be able to offer a name of a lawyer who they suggest you reach out to. They may do this even if the topic has little to do with their specific area of expertise or the area of focus of that organization.

Some organizations listed here will fully embrace the right case and will go so far as to fully fund resolution of the legal matter. Simply picking up the phone and reaching out to a likeminded person can go a long way in helping you resolve any legal concerns you have.

You are not alone. There are many resources available to you, but they will never knock on your door insisting you pursue justice. You must be the actor in your life. You must be the actor in order for your injustice to reach a more justice resolution. That means doggedly seeking a solution and being determined to communicate properly to those in a position to magnify your efforts and provide assistance. In this list and the next you will find a good starting place.

Alabama
Free the People
611 Pennsylvania Ave #259
Washington, DC 20003
312-835-6431
freethepeople.org

Principles That Matter
2770 Arapahoe Rd
Suite 132-116
Lafayette, CO 80026
720-903-3737
principlesthatmatter.org

Alabama Policy Institute
2213 Morris Ave First Floor
Birmingham, AL 35203
205-870-9900
alabamapolicy.org

Alaska
Alaska Policy Forum
7926 Old Seward Hwy
Suite A6
Anchorage, AK 99518
907-334-5853
alaskapolicyforum.org

Arizona
American Juris Link
7000 N 16 St Suite 120-155
Phoenix, AZ 85020
703-243-1655
americanjurislink.org

Goldwater Institute
500 E. Coronado Road
Phoenix, AZ 85004
602-462-5000
goldwaterinstitute.org

Alliance for
Defending Freedom
15100 N. 90th Street
Scottsdale, AZ 85260
480-444-0020
adflegal.org

Arkansas
Advance Arkansas Institute
55 Fontenay Circle Little
Rock, AR 72223
501-588-4245
advancearkansas.org

Arkansas Policy Foundation
111 Center Street
Suite 1200
Little Rock, AR 72201
501-537-0825
arkansaspolicyfoundation.org

California
California Policy Center
18002 Irvine Blvd
Suite 108
Tustin, CA 92780
714-714-8871
californiapolicycenter.org

Freedom Foundation
PO Box 6683
Fullerton, CA 92834
949-954-8914
freedomfoundation.com

Pacific Research Institute
PO Box 60485
Pasadena, CA 91116
415-989-0833
pacificresearch.org

Pacific Justice Institute
P.O. Box 276600
Sacramento, CA 95827-6600
916-857-6900
pacificjustice.org

The Freedom of Conscience
Defense Fund
16236 San Dieguito Rd
Bldg. 3, Suite #3-15
Rancho Santa Fe, CA 92091
858-759-9948
fcdflegal.org

Barnes Law
601 South Figueroa Street
Suite 4050
Los Angeles, CA 90017
213-330-3341
barneslawllp.com

For Kids & Country
2518 Via Durazno
San Clemente, CA 92673
714-421-0892
forkidsandcountry.org

Independent Institute
100 Swan Way
Oakland, CA 94621
510-632-1366
independent.org

Lincoln Network
2443 Fillmore St 380-3386
San Francisco, CA 94115
703-243-1655
joinlincoln.org

National Tax
Limitation Committee
1700 Eureka Rd
Suite 150A
Roseville, CA
916-786-9400
limittaxes.org

Pacific Legal Foundation
930 G Street
Sacramento, CA 95814
916-419-7111
pacificlegal.org

Reason Foundation
5737 Mesmer Ave
Los Angeles, CA 90230
310-391-2245
reason.org

Colorado
Centennial Institute
8787 W Alameda Ave
Lakewood, CO 80226
303-963-3424
ccu.edu

Leadership Program
of the Rockies
1777 South Harrison Street
Suite 807
Denver, CO 80210
303-488-0018
leadershipprogram.org

Mountain States
Legal Foundation
2596 S Lewis Way
Lakewood, CO 80227
303-292-2021
mslegal.org

Steamboat Institute
27855 Whitewood Drive
East Steamboat Springs, CO
80487
970-846-6013
steamboatinstitute.org

Independence Institute
727 E. 16th Ave
Denver, CO 80203
303-279-6536
i2i.org

Connecticut
Yankee Institute
for Public Policy
216 Main Street
Hartford, NH 06106
860-282-0722
yankeeinstitute.org

Delaware
Intercollegiate
Studies Institute
3901 Centerville Road
Wilmington, DE 19807
800-526-7022
isi.org

Caesar Rodney Institute
420 Corporate Blvd
Newark, DE 19702
302-273-0080
caesarrodney.org

Florida
ExcelinEd
P.O. Box 10691
Tallahassee, FL 32302
850-391-4090
excelined.org

Foundation for
Government Accountability
15275 Collier Blvd
Suite 201-279
Naples, FL 34119
239-244-8808
thefga.org

James Madison Institute
100 North Duval Street
Tallahassee, FL 32301
850-386-3131
jamesmadison.org

Liberty Counsel
PO Box 540774
Orlando, FL 32854
407-875-1776
lc.org

Georgia

Foundation for
Economic Education
1819 Peachtree Road NE
Suite 300
Atlanta, GA 30309
404-554-9980
fee.org

Georgia Center
for Opportunity
333 Research Court
Suite 210
Peachtree Corners, GA 30092
770-242-0001
georgiaopportunity.org

Georgia Public
Policy Foundation
3200 Cobb Galleria Parkway
Suite 214
Atlanta, GA 30339
404-256-4050
georgiapolicy.org

Southeastern
Legal Foundation
560 West Crossville Rd
Suite 104
Roswell, GA 30075
770-977-2131
slfliberty.org

Hawaii

Grassroot Institute of Hawaii
1050 Bishop St 508
Honolulu, HI 96813
808-591-9193
grassrootinstitute.org

Idaho

Idaho Freedom Foundation
802 W Bannock St Suite 405
Boise, ID 83702
208-258-2280
idahofreedom.org

Illinois

Illinois Policy Institute
190 South LaSalle St
Suite 1500
Chicago, IL 60603
312-346-5700
illinoispolicy.org

Think Freely Media
190 S. LaSalle St
Suite 1500
Chicago, IL 60603
202-838-3175
thinkfreelymedia.org

Heartland Institute
3939 North Wilke Road
Arlington Heights, IL 60004
312-377-4000
heartland.org

Liberty Justice Center
190 S La Salle St
Suite 1500
Chicago, IL 60603-3410
312-263-7668
libertyjusticecenter.org

The Policy Circle
1189 Wilmette Ave #210
Wilmette, IL 60091
847-906-3350
thepolicycircle.org

Indiana
EdChoice
111 Monument Circle
Suite 2650
Indianapolis, IN 46204
317-681-0745
edchoice.org

Indiana Policy
Review Foundation
P.O. Box 5166
Fort Wayne, IN 46895
260-417-4094
inpolicy.org

The James Madison Center
1 South 6th Street,
Terre Haute, IN 47807
812-232-2434
jamesmadisoncenter.org

Iowa
Tax Education Foundation
9295 Bishop Drive #105
West Des Moines, IA 50266
563-264-8080
taxeducationfoundation.org

Kansas
Kansas Policy Institute
250 N. Water St.
Wichita, KS 67202
316-634-0218
kansaspolicy.org

Kentucky
Bluegrass Institute
P.O. Box 11706
Lexington, KY 40577
859-444-5630
bipps.org

Pegasus Institute
235 S. 5th Street
Louisville, KY 40202
270-617-3627
pegasuskentucky.org

Louisiana
Louisiana Family Forum
655 St. Ferdinand Street
Baton Rouge, LA 70802
225-344-8533
lafamilyforum.org

Pelican Institute
for Public Policy
400 Poydras
Suite 900
New Orleans, LA 70130
504-500-0506
pelicaninstitute.org

Maine
Maine Policy Institute
P.O. Box 7829
Portland, ME 04112
207-321-2550
mainepolicy.org

Maryland
Free State Foundation
6259 Executive Blvd
Rockville, MD 20852
301-984-8253
freestatefoundation.org

The Maryland Public
Policy Institute
One Research Court
Suite 450
Rockville, MD 20850
240-686-3510
mdpolicy.org

Massachusetts
Beacon Hill Institute for
Public Policy Research
165 Main Street
Suite 306
Medway, MA 02053
855-244-4550
beaconhill.org

Pioneer Institute
185 Devonshire Street
Unit 1101
Boston, MA 02110
617-723-2277
pioneerinstitute.org

Michigan
Acton Institute
98 E. Fulton Street
Grand Rapids, MI 49503
616-454-3080
acton.org

The Thomas More Law Center
24 Frank Lloyd Wright Drive
P.O. Box 393
Ann Arbor, MI 48106
734-827-2001
thomasmore.org

The College Fix
P.O. Box 76
Hillsdale, MI 49242
760-809-5715
thecollegefix.com

Mackinac Center
for Public Policy
P.O. Box 568
140 West Main Street
Midland, MI 48640
989-631-0900
mackinac.org

Minnesota
Center of the
American Experiment
8441 Wayzata Blvd
Suite 350
Golden Valley, MN 55426
612-338-3605
americanexperiment.org

Freedom Foundation
of Minnesota
825 Nicollet Mall
Suite 815
Minneapolis, MN 55402
612-354-2160
freedomfoundation.
publishpath.com

Mississippi
Empower Mississippi
Foundation
1000 Northpark Dr
Ridgeland, MS 39157
601-980-1897
empowerms.org

Mississippi Center
for Public Policy
520 George Street
Jackson, MS 39202
601-969-1300
mspolicy.org

Missouri
Freedom Center of Missouri
14779 Audrain Rd. 815
Mexico, MO 65265
573-567-0307
mofreedom.org

Show-Me Institute
5297 Washington Place
Saint Louis, MO 63108
816-561-1777
showmeinstitute.org

Montana
Property & Environment
Research Center
2048 Analysis Dr
Suite A
Bozeman, MT 59718
406-587-9591
perc.org

Montana Policy Institute
PO Box 852
Helena, MT 59601
406-480-1269
montanapolicy.org

Nebraska
Platte Institute for
Economic Research
6910 Pacific St
Suite 216
Omaha, NE 68106
402-452-3737
platteinstitute.org

Nevada
Nevada Policy
Research Institute
7130 Placid St.
Las Vegas, NV 89119
702-222-0642
npri.org

New Hampshire
Granite Institute
P.O. Box 125
Woodsville, NH 03785
603-728-8257
graniteinstitute.org

Josiah Bartlett Center
for Public Policy
P.O. Box 897
Concord, NH 03302
603-715-0076
jbartlett.org

New Jersey
Garden State Initiative
12 Quimby Lane
Bernardsville, NJ 07924
908-400-9688
gardenstateinitiative.org

New Mexico
Rio Grande Foundation
PO Box 40336
Albuquerque, NM 87196
505-264-6090
riograndefoundation.org

New York
American Civil Liberties Union
125 Broad Street, 18th Floor
New York, NY 10004
212-549-2500
aclu.org

Manhattan Institute
for Policy Research
52 Vanderbilt Ave Third Floor
New York, NY 10017
212-599-7000
manhattan-institute.org

National Review Institute
19 W 44th Street
Suite 1701
New York, NY 10036
212-849-2806
nrinstitute.org

Empire Center
for Public Policy
30 South Pearl Street
Suite 1210
Albany, NY 12207
518-434-3100
empirecenter.org

North Carolina
Jesse Helms Center
Post Office Box 247
Wingate, NC 28174-0247
704-233-1776
jessehelmscenter.org

The James G. Martin Center
for Academic Renewal
353 E. Six Forks Road
Suite 200
Raleigh, NC 27609
919-828-1400
jamesgmartin.center

Civitas Institute
805 Spring Forest Road
Suite 100
Raleigh, NC 27609
919-747-8061
nccivitas.org

John Locke Foundation
4800 Six Forks Rd
Suite 220
Raleigh, NC 27609
919-828-3876
johnlocke.org

North Dakota
Roughrider Policy Center
820 34th Ave E
Suite 200
West Fargo, ND 58078
701-354-3934
roughriderpolicy.org

Ohio
1851 Center for
Constitutional Law
122 E Main Street
Fourth Floor
Columbus, OH 43215
614-340-9817
ohioconstitution.org

Ashbrook Center
401 College Ave
Ashland, OH 44805
419-289-5411
ashbrook.org

Forge Leadership Network
707 Miamisburg
-Centerville Rd
Dayton, OH 45459
800-481-5024
forgeleadership.org

Freedom Foundation (Ohio)
P.O. Box 16309
Columbus, OH 43216
567-214-6355
freedomfoundation.com

The Buckeye Institute
88 East Broad Street
Suite 1300
Columbus, OH 43215
614-224-4422
buckeyeinstitute.org

Oklahoma
1889 Institute
1401 N. Lincoln Blvd
Suite 175
Oklahoma City, OK 73104
405-646-3272
1889institute.org

EFoundation
2 East California Ave
Oklahoma City, OK 73104
405-646-3465
efoundationok.org

Oklahoma Council
of Public Affairs
1401 N Lincoln Blvd
Oklahoma City, OK 73104
405-602-1667
ocpathink.org

Oregon
Cascade Policy Institute
4850 SW Scholls Ferry Road
Suite 103
Portland, OR 97225
503-242-0900
cascadepolicy.org

Freedom Foundation
(Oregon)
PO Box 18146
Salem, OR 97305
503-951-6208
freedomfoundation.com

Pennsylvania
Center for
Independent Thought
1420 Walnut Street,
Suite 1011
Philadelphia, PA 19102
215-546-0501
centerforindependent
thought.org

Free To Choose Network
2002 Filmore Ave
Erie, PA 16506
814-833-7140
freetochoosenetwork.org

Freedoms Foundation
at Valley Forge
1601 Valley Forge Rd
Valley Forge, PA 19481
800-896-5488
freedomsfoundation.org

Commonwealth Foundation
for Public Policy Alternatives
225 State Street
Suite 302
Harrisburg, PA 17101
717-671-1901
commonwealth
foundation.org

Freedom Foundation
(Pennsylvania)
P.O. Box 1069
Kennett Square, PA 19348
484-747-6072
freedomfoundation.com

Rhode Island
Rhode Island Center for
Freedom and Prosperity
P.O. Box 10069
Cranston, RI 02910
401-429-6115
rifreedom.org

South Carolina
Center for
Independent Employees
PO Box 2421
Spartanburg, SC 29304
864-316-9050
centerforindependent
employees.org

Palmetto Promise Institute
P.O. Box 12676
Columbia, SC 29211
803-708-0673
palmettopromise.org

South Dakota
Great Plains Public
Policy Institute
P.O. Box 88138
Sioux Falls, SD 57109-8138
605-334-9400
greatplainsppi.org

Tennessee
Beacon Center of Tennessee
201 4th Ave North
Suite 1820
Nashville, TN 37219
615-383-6431
beacontn.org

Texas
First Liberty Institute
2001 West Plano Parkway
Suite 1600
Plano, TX 75075
972-941-4444
firstliberty.org

Benjamin Rush Institute
8610 Glenmont Street North
Richland Hills, TX 76182
214-507-4610
benjaminrushinstitute.org

Lone Star Policy Institute
8390 Lyndon B Johnson
Freeway, Suite 570
Dallas, TX 75243
214-800-5590
lonestarpolicyinstitute.org

The Foundation for
Research on Equal
Opportunity
201 W Fifth Street
Suite 1100
Austin, TX 78701
512-537-1070
freopp.org

Texas Public
Policy Foundation
901 Congress Ave
Austin, TX 78701
512-472-2700
texaspolicy.com

Utah
Center for Growth
and Opportunity at
Utah State University
3525 Old Main Hill
Logan, UT 84322
435-557-0795
thecgo.org

Next Generation
Freedom Fund
1737 Wood Glen Rd
Sandy, UT 84092
385-202-5050
transcendtogether.org

Libertas Institute
2183 W Main St
Suite A102
Lehi, UT 84043
801-901-0310
libertasutah.org

Sutherland Institute
15 West South Temple
Suite 200
Salt Lake City, UT 84101
801-355-1272
sutherlandinstitute.org

Vermont

Ethan Allen Institute
36 Owls Head Lane
Stowe, VT 05672
802-695-1448
ethanallen.org

Virginia

America's Future Foundation
3434 Washington Blvd
1st Floor
Arlington, VA 22201
202-331-2261
americasfuture.org

American Conservative
Union Foundation
1199 N Fairfax St
Suite 500
Alexandria, VA 22314
202-347-9388
conservative.org

American Legislative
Exchange Council
2900 Crystal Drive
Suite 600
Arlington, VA 22202
703-373-0933
alec.org

Americans for Fair Treatment
225 State Street
Suite 301
Harrisburg, PA 17101
717-216-4756
americansforfairtreatment.org

Americans for Prosperity
1310 N Courthouse Rd
Suite 700
Arlington, VA 22201
703-224-3200
americansforprosperity
foundation.org

Association of American
Educators Foundation
2560 Huntington Ave
Suite 301
Alexandria, VA 22303
703-739-2100
aaeteachers.org

Atlas Network
4075 Wilson Blvd
Suite 310
Arlington, VA 22203
202-449-8449
atlasnetwork.org

Bill of Rights Institute
1310 North Courthouse Road
Suite 620
Arlington, VA 22201
703-894-1776
billofrightsinstitute.org

Charles Koch Institute
1320 N. Courthouse Road
Suite 500
Arlington, VA 22201
703-875-1770
charleskochfoundation.org

DonorsTrust
1800 Diagonal Rd
Suite 280
Alexandria, VA 22314
703-535-3563
donorstrust.org

Energy & Environment
Legal Institute
1350 Beverly Rd
Suite 115-445
McLean, VA 22101
202-810-2001
eelegal.org

Franklin News Foundation
200 West Madison Street
Suite 2100
Chicago, IL 60606
847-497-5230
franklinnews.org

Galen Institute
PO Box 130 Paeonian
Springs, VA 20129
703-687-4665
galen.org

Institute for Family Studies
P.O. Box 7967
Charlottesville, VA 22906
434-260-1770
ifstudies.org

Institute for Free Speech
1150 Connecticut Ave, NW
Suite 801
Washington, DC 20036
202-301-3300
ifs.org

Institute for Humane Studies
3434 Washington Blvd
1st Floor
Arlington, VA 22201
703-993-4880
theihs.org

Institute for Justice
901 N. Glebe Road
Suite 900
Arlington, VA 22203
703-682-9320
ij.org

Landmark Legal Foundation
19415 Deerfield Ave
Suite 312
Leesburg, VA 20176
703-554-6100
landmarklegal.org

Leadership Institute
Steven P.J. Wood Building
1101 North Highland Street
Arlington, VA 22201
703-247-2000
leadershipinstitute.org

Mercatus Center at
George Mason University
3434 Washington Blvd
4th Floor
Arlington, VA 22201
703-993-4930
mercatus.org

National Right to Work
Legal Defense &
Education Foundation Inc.
8001 Braddock Road
Suite 600
Springfield, VA 22160
800-336-3600
nrtw.org

Prison Fellowship
44180 Riverside Parkway
Lansdowne, VA 20176
800-206-9764
prisonfellowship.org

Young America's Foundation
11480 Commerce Park Dr
Suite 600
Reston, VA 20191
703-318-9608
yaf.org

State Policy Network
1655 N Fort Myer Dr
Suite 360
Arlington, VA 22209
703-243-1655
spn.org

Students For Liberty
2221 S Clark St 12th Floor
Arlington, VA 22202
202-733-2409
studentsforliberty.org

Thomas Jefferson Institute
for Public Policy
7011 Dreams Way Court
Alexandria, VA 22315
703-440-9447
thomasjeffersoninst.org

The Center for
American Liberty
PO Box 2510
Leesburg, VA 20177
703-687-6212
libertycenter.org

The Rutherford Institute
Post Office Box 7482
Charlottesville, VA 22906
434-978-3888
rutherford.org

Virginia Institute
for Public Policy
P.O. Box 1123
Abingdon, VA 24212
540-245-1776
virginiainstitute.org

Washington
Freedom Foundation
(Washington)
PO Box 552
Olympia, WA 98507-0552
360-956-3482
freedomfoundation.com

Washington Policy Center
PO Box 3643
Seattle, WA 98124
206-937-9691
washingtonpolicy.org

Washington DC

American Council of
Trustees and Alumni
1730 M Street NW
Suite 600
Washington, DC 20036
202-467-6787
goacta.org

The First Amendment
Lawyers Association
1201 Connecticut Ave NW
#500B
Washington, DC 20036
202-540-9817
firstamendmentlawyers.org

American Enterprise Institute
1789 Massachusetts Ave NW
Washington, DC 20036
202-862-5800
aei.org

Americans for Tax Reform
722 12th Street NW 4th Floor
Washington, DC 20005
202-785-0266
atr.org

Archbridge Institute
810 7th Street NE
Washington, DC 20002
202-486-8457
archbridgeinstitute.org

Becket
1200 New Hampshire
Ave NW Suite 700
Washington, DC 20036
202-955-0095
becketlaw.org

Capital Research Center
1513 16th Street NW
Washington, DC 20036
202-483-6900
capitalresearch.org

Cato Institute
1000 Massachusetts Ave NW
Washington, DC 20001
202-842-0200
cato.org

Center for Education Reform
1455 Pennsylvania Ave NW
Suite 250
Washington, DC 20004
202-750-0016
edreform.com

Citizens Against
Government Waste
1100 Connecticut Ave NW
Suite 650
Washington, DC 20036
202-467-5300
cagw.org

Competitive
Enterprise Institute
1310 L Street NW 7th floor
Washington, DC 20005
202-331-1010
cei.org

Federalist Society
1776 I Street NW
Suite 300
Washington, DC 20006
202-822-8138
fedsoc.org

FreedomWorks
111 K Street NE
Suite 600
Washington, DC 20002
202-783-3870
freedomworks.org

Heritage Foundation
214 Massachusetts Ave NE
Washington, DC 20002
202-546-4400
heritage.org

Independent Women's Forum
1875 I Street NW
Suite 500
Washington, DC 20006
202-857-5201
iwf.org

Judicial Watch
425 Third Street SW
Suite 800
Washington, DC 20024
202-646-5172
judicialwatch.org

National Taxpayers
Union Foundation
122 C Street NW
Suite 650
Washington, DC 20001
703-683-5700
ntu.org

New Civil Liberties Alliance
1225 19th Street NW
Suite 450
Washington, DC 20036
202-869-5210
nclalegal.org

Philanthropy Roundtable
1120 20th Street NW
Suite 550S
Washington, DC 20036
202-822-8333
philanthropyroundtable.org

R Street Institute
1212 New York Ave NW
Suite 900
Washington, DC 20005
202-525-5717
rstreet.org

Speech First
1300 I St NW
Suite 400E
Washington, DC 20005
571-766-6883
speechfirst.org

Tax Foundation
1325 G Street NW
Suite 950
Washington, DC 20005
202-464-6200
taxfoundation.org

The American
Consumer Institute
1701 Pennsylvania Ave NW
Suite 200
Washington, DC 20006
703-282-9400
theamericanconsumer.org

The Fund for
American Studies
1706 New Hampshire Ave
Washington, DC 20009
202-986-0384
tfas.org

Young Voices
1342 Florida Ave NW
Washington, DC 20009
571-289-8904
young-voices.com

West Virginia
Cardinal Institute
P.O. Box 11495
Charleston, WV 25339
304-881-1012
cardinalinstitute.com

Wisconsin
Badger Institute
700 W. Virginia Street
Suite 301
Milwaukee, WI 53204
414-225-9940
badgerinstitute.org

MacIver Institute
for Public Policy
10 E. Doty Street
Suite 820
Madison, WI 53703
608-588-6477
maciverinstitute.com

Wisconsin Institute
for Law & Liberty
330 East Kilbourn Ave
Suite 725
Milwaukee, WI 53202
414-727-9455
will-law.org

Lucy Burns Institute
8383 Greenway Blvd
Suite 600
Middleton, WI 53562
608-255-0688
balotpedia.org/Lucy_Burns
_Institute

School Choice Wisconsin
350 Bishops Way
Suite 104
Brookfield, WI 53005
414-319-9160
schoolchoicewi.org

Wyoming
Wyoming Liberty Group
1902 Thomes Ave
Suite 201A
Cheyenne, WY 82001
307-632-7020
wyliberty.org

The Block List

In the American legal system, non-lawyers are effectively second-class citizens.

One need only enter the front door of many courthouses to be made aware of that detail, as one security line exists for lawyers and a second for all others. Even deeper in the legal system, this distinction is painfully apparent.

Some people may not travel in the circles needed to access first class representation.

This is a list made with the intent of putting greater first-class representation in the hands of people with the right philosophical ideas and the right amount of passion to make such a list meaningful, the readers of these pages.

In 2012, Loyola University Professor Walter Block answered the question "Who would be a fitting Supreme Court Justice under a Ron Paul presidency?"

Walter Block made a list and returned to it several times to add to it.

To be Blocklisted as an attorney is a great honor and says a great deal about ones sense of professional integrity.

As the United States turns its attention to the Supreme Court, as is done in every election year, The Block List could perhaps use a refresh of the latest attorneys that appear on that list.

For the first time ever, here is a collection of publicly available contact information for every member of The 2012 Block List.

It is here assembled as a resource for those who would do good with it by reaching out to the lawyers listed here and asking them to aid you in a pressing legal matter of public importance, either in their direct service, or by asking them to tap their networks for aide.

Jonathan Adler
Case Western
Reserve University
George Gund Hall
11075 East Blvd
Cleveland, OH 44106
(216) 368-3600
jonathan.adler@case.edu

Avril Allen
65 Queen Street West
Suite 1000
Toronto, Ontario, M5H 2M5
Canada
(416) 367-5558 ext. 212

Paul Aubert
550 Club Dr
Suite 445
Montgomery, TX 77316-3096
(713) 516-2670
paubert@me.com

Steve Bainbridge
UCLA School of Law
385 Charles E. Young Dr. East
Los Angeles, CA 90095
bainbridge@law.ucla.edu

Daren Bakst
3003 Van Ness St NW
Washington, DC 20008-4701
(202) 546-4400

Randy Barnett
Georgetown Law
600 New Jersey Ave NW
Washington, DC 20001
(202) 662-9936
rb325@law.georgetown.edu

William Barnett II
Loyola University
New Orleans
College of Business
6363 St. Charles Ave
Campus Box 172
New Orleans, LA 70118
(504) 864-7950
wbarnett@loyno.edu

Jeffrey Barr
Armstrong Teasdale
3770 Howard Hughes
Parkway, Suite 200
Las Vegas, NV 89169
(702) 678-5070
jbarr@atllp.com

Joe Becker
Mises Institute
518 West Magnolia Avenue
Auburn, Alabama 36832-4501
(334) 321-2100
becker@mises.org

Stuart Benjamin
Duke University School of Law
210 Science Dr
Durham, NC 27708
(919) 613-7275
benjamin@law.duke.edu

Shana Black
8880 Rio San Diego Drive
Suite 800
San Diego, CA 92108
(619) 557-0122
shana@shanablack.com

Clint Bolick
Arizona Supreme Court
1501 W Washington
Phoenix, AZ 85007
(602) 452-3300

Don Boudreaux
George Mason University
4400 University Drive, 3G4
Fairfax, VA 22030
(703) 993-1151
dboudrea@gmu.edu

Walter Boytinck
4388 Pine Crescent
Vancouver, BC V6J 4L1
Canada

Janice Rogers Brown
E. Barrett Prettyman
United States Courthouse
333 Constitution Ave NW
Fifth Floor, Room 5205
Washington, DC 20001
(202) 216-7220

Scott Bullock
Institute for Justice
901 N. Glebe Road
Suite 900
Arlington, VA 22203
(703) 682-9320
sbullock@ij.org

Gary Chartier
La Sierra University
4500 Riverwalk Parkway
Riverside, CA 92505
(951) 785-2181
gchartie@lasierra.edu

Max Chiz
(504) 383-4629
office@electchiz.com

Dick Clark
Dick Clark Law
1028 G Street
Suite 105
Lincoln, NE 68508
(402) 915-1791
dick@dickclarklaw.com

Mila Cobanov-Vecore
960 21st St., Apt. F
Santa Monica, CA 90403
(248) 631-9374

Ronald Coffey
Case Western
Reserve University
10900 Euclid Ave
Cleveland, OH 44106
(216) 368-2000
rjc4@case.edu

Lloyd Cohen
George Mason University
3301 Fairfax Dr
Arlington, VA 22201
(703) 993-8048
lcohen2@gmu.edu

Jeff Deist
Mises Institute
518 West Magnolia Ave
Auburn, AL 36832-4501
(334) 321-2100
jeffdeist@mises.org

David Deiteman
Penn State Behrend
281 Burke Center
Erie, PA 16563
(814) 898-6506
dfd12@psu.edu

John Denson
Mises Institute
West Magnolia Ave
Auburn, AL 36832-4501
(334) 321-2100

George Dent
Case Western
Reserve University
10900 Euclid Ave
Cleveland, OH 44106
(213) 368-3311
george.dent@case.edu

Steven Eagle
Antonin Scalia Law School
George Mason University
3301 Fairfax Dr
Arlington, VA 22201
(703) 993-8030
seagle@gmu.edu

Brad Edmonds
GSB Incorporated
3555 NW 58th Street,
Suite 700W
Oklahoma City, OK 73112
(405) 848-9549
gsb@gsb-inc.com

Richard Epstein
New York University
School of Law
40 Washington Sq. South
New York, NY 10012
(212) 992-8858
richard.epstein@nyu.edu

Robert Fast
The Fast Law Firm
6278 North Federal
Highway, Suite #237
Fort Lauderdale, FL 33308
(954) 324-7529
info@thefastlawfirm.com

Bruce Fein
Bruce Fein Law
910 Seventeenth Street NW
Suite 800
Washington, DC 20006
(202) 775-1787

Tiffany Fleming
Butler Law Firm
2400 Veterans Blvd
Suite 485
Kenner, LA 70062
(504) 305-4117

Deanna Forbush French
Fox Rothschild
1980 Festival Plaza Drive
Suite 700
Las Vegas, NV 89135
(702) 699-5169

Derek From
Canadian
Constitution Foundation
6025 - 12 St SE
Suite 215
Calgary, AB T2H 2K1 Canada
(888) 695-9105
derek.james.from@gmail.com

Martin Fronek
White and Case LLP
Na Prikope 14
110 00 Nove Mesto
Czech Republic
+420 255-771-111
mfronek@whitecase.com

Eric Gookin
321 E 12th St.
Des Moines, IA 50319-1002
(515) 281-7550

David Gruning
Loyola University
New Orleans
College of Law
7214 St. Charles Ave
Campus Box 901
New Orleans, LA 70118
(504) 861-5653
gruning@loyno.edu

Kevin Gutzman
Department of History
Western Connecticut
State University
181 White Street
Danbury, CT 06810
gutzmank@wcsu.edu

John Hasnas
Georgetown Law
600 New Jersey Avenue
Washington DC 20001
(202) 687-4825
hasnasj@georgetown.edu

Jared Hausmann
Simmons Hanly Conroy
One Court Street
Alton, IL 62002
(618) 693-3104
jhausmann@simmonsfirm.com

Thomas Hazlett
Clemson University
233 Sirrine Hall
Clemson University
225 Walter T. Cox Blvd
Clemson, SC 29634
(864) 656-3481
hazlett@clemson.edu

Gene Healy
Cato Institute
1000 Massachusetts Ave NW
Washington DC 20001
(202) 789-5200
ghealy@cato.org

Jule Herbert
Herbert Law Firm
218 Professional Court
Gulf Shores, AL 36547
(251) 968-4764

Christopher Homer
Competitive
Enterprise Institute
1310 L Street NW
7th Floor
Washington, DC 20005
(202) 331-1010
info@cei.org

Jacob Hornberger
The Future
of Freedom Foundation
11350 Random Hills Road
Suite 800
Fairfax, VA 22030
(703) 934-6101
jhornberger@fff.org

Jacob Huebert
Mises Institute
518 West Magnolia Ave
Auburn, AL 36832-4501
(334) 321-2100
jhhuebert@gmail.com

Christine Hurt
Brigham Young University
J. Reuben Clark Building
Brigham Young University
Provo, UT 84602
(801) 422-5354
hurtc@law.byu.edu

Lee Iglody
Iglody Law
7450 Arroyo Crossing Pkwy
Suite 270
Las Vegas, NV 89113
(702) 425-5366
lee@iglody.com

Stavros Katsios
GeoLab Institute
7 Tsirigoti Sq
GR-49132
Corfu, Greece
+30-26610-87238
director@geolabinstitute.org

Sam Kazman
Competitive
Enterprise Institute
1310 L Street NW
7th Floor
Washington, DC 20005
(202) 331-1010
sam.kazman@cei.org

Stephan Kinsella
3101 Avalon Pl.
Houston, TX 77019
(713) 416-0006
nkinsella@gmail.com

Manuel S. Klausner
Klausner Law Offices
5538 Red Oak Dr
Los Angeles, CA 90068-2551
(213) 617-0414
MKlausner@klausnerlaw.us

Russell Korobkin
UCLA School of Law
385 Charles E. Young Dr. East
Los Angeles, CA 90095
(310) 825-1994
korobkin@law.ucla.edu

Michael Krauss
Antonin Scalia Law School
George Mason University
3301 Fairfax Dr
Arlington, VA 22201
(703) 993-8024
mkrauss@gmu.edu

Thomas Lambert
Lambert Law
P.O. Box 22530
San Diego, CA 92192
(858) 452-2000
thl@san.rr.com

Jamie Ianelli
5444 57th Ave. S
Seattle, WA, 98118
(206) 384-2400
jamesianelli@gmail.com

Christie LaPorte
Galloway Johnson,
Tompkins, Burr and Smith
#3 Sanctuary Boulevard
Suite 301
Mandeville, LA 70471
(958) 674-6680
claporte@gjtbs.com

Bart Lee
Spiegel Liao &Kagay
388 Market Street
Suite 900
San Francisco, CA 94111
(415) 956-5959
blee@slksf.com

George Leef
James G. Martin Center
for Academic Renewal
353 E. Six Forks Road
Suite 200
Raleigh, NC 27609
(919) 828-1400
georgeleef@popecenter.org

Glen Lenihan
Oved & Oved Attorneys
401 Greenwich Street
New York, NY 10013
(212) 226-2376
glenihan@ovedlaw.com

Dan Levine
Cozen O'Connor
One Liberty Place
1650 Market St
Suite 2800
Philadelphia, PA 19103
(215) 864-8047
dlevin@cozen.com

Robert Levy
Procopio Attorney
525 B Street
Suite 2200
San Diego, CA 92101
(619) 515-3243
robert.levy@procopio.com

Floy Lilly
Mises Institute
518 West Magnolia Avenue
Auburn, AL 36832-4501
(334) 321-2155
floylilley@bellsouth.net

Mike Lloyd
Covington & Burling LLP
One City Center
850 Tenth St NW
Washington, DC 20001-4956
(202) 662-5343
mlloyd@cov.com

Jonathan R. Macey
Yale Law School
127 Wall Street
New Haven, CT 06511
(203) 432-7913
jonathan.macey@yale.edu

Gary Mah
Sporer Mah & Co.
Tri-City Business Centre
#2300-2850 Shaughnessy St
Port Coquitlam, BC V3C 6K5
Canada
(604) 717-5510
gmah@sporermah.com

Geoffrey Manne
International Center
for Law & Economics
1104 NW 15th Ave
Suite 300
Portland, OR 97209
gmanne@laweconcenter.org

Kevin A. McCabe
Dickinson Public
Defender Office
135 Sims St., Ste. 221
Dickinson, ND 58601
(701) 227-7460
kmccabe@nd.gov

Todd McMullan
Fried Frank
One New York Plaza
New York, NY 10004
(212) 859-8190
todd.mcmullan
@friedfrank.com

William Mellor
Institute For Justice
901 N Glebe Rd
Suite 900
Arlington, VA, 22203
(703) 682-9320
wmellor@ij.org

Andrei Mincov
Mincov Law Corporation
300 — 1055 W. Hastings St
Vancouver, BC V6E 2E9
Canada
(778) 869-7281
andrei@mincovlaw.com

Joe Morrel
Porter Hedges
1000 Main St., 36th Floor
Houston, TX 77002
(713) 226-6606
jmorrel@porterhedges.com

Andrew Morriss
Linklaters
1290 Avenue of the Americas
New York, NY 10104
(212) 903-9048
andrew.morris@linklaters.com

Andrew Napolitano
Mintz & Gold LLP
600 Third Avenue
25th Floor
New York, NY 10016
(212) 696-4848
napolitano
@mintzandgold.com

Nadia Nedzel
Southern University
2 Roosevelt Steptoe Drive
Baton Rounge, LA 70813
(225) 771-4900 ext. 221
nnedzel@sulc.edu

Clark Neily
Cato Institute
1000 Massachusetts Ave NW
Washington, DC 20001-5403
(202) 842-0200
cneily@cato.org

Michael O'Brian
Auckland, New Zealand
P.O. Box 4006
Shortland Street
Auckland, 1140, New Zealand
(642)138-0273
michael@michaelobrien.co.nz

James Ostrowski
63 Newport Ave.
Buffalo, NY 14216-1508
 (716) 435-8918
jameso@apollo3.com

David Post
David Post Law Firm
1411 W Innes St
Salisbury, NC 28144
(704) 267-7000
david@davidpostlaw.com

Todd Ptak
Airbus Group Sas
B80 Building 2
Rond-Point Dewoitine
BP 90112
31703 Blagnac Cedex
France
+33 581 31 7500

Glenn Reynolds
The University
of Tennessee, Knoxville
Knoxville, TN 37996
(865) 974-1000
greynold@utk.edu

Stewart Rhodes
info@oathkeepers.org

Greg Rome
Greg Rome Attorney at Law
201 Napoleon Street
Baton Rouge, LA 70802
(225) 248-1234
greg.rome@romelawbr.com

Roger Roots
Lysander Spooner University
113 Lake Drive East
Livingston, MT 59047
(406) 224-3105
rogerroots@msn.com

Clay Rossi
P.O. Box 2481
Mobile, AL 36652
(251) 574-3400

Noah D. Rubins
Freshfields
Bruckhaus Deringer
2 rue Paul Cezanne
75008 Paris, France
+33 1 44 56 44 56
noah.rubins@freshfields.com

Ron Rychlak
The University of Mississippi
School of Law
481 Chucky Mullins Drive
University, MS 38677
(662) 915-6841
rrychlak@olemiss.edu

Sukrit Sabhlok
Macquarie University
Law School
6 First Walk
Sydney, New South Wales
2109 Australia
sukrit.sabhlok
@students.mq.edu.au

Matt Saltzman
Saltzman Mugan Dushoff
1835 Village Center Circle
Las Vegas, NV 89134
(702) 405-8500
msaltzman
@nvbusinesslaw.com

Emmanouil Savoidakis
Polis and Partners Law Firm
14, Solonos St
GR 106 73, Athens, Greece
+30 210 7297252
esavoidakis@politispartners.gr

Chris Schafer
16000 North Dallas Pkwy
Suite 550
Dallas, TX 75248
(469) 766-7881
chris.schafer@gmail.com

Karen Selick
kas@karenselick.com

Ilya Shapiro
Cato Institute
1000 Massachusetts Ave NW
Washington, DC 20001-5403
(202) 789-5200
ishapiro@cato.org

Keith Sharfman
St. John's University
School of Law
8000 Utopia Parkway
Queens, NY 11439
(718) 990-6600
sharfmak@stjohns.edu

Paul Sherman
Institute for Justice
901 N. Glebe Road
Suite 900
Arlington, VA 22203
(703) 682-9320
psherman@ij.org

Norman Singleton
Campaign for Liberty
5211 Port Royal Road
Suite 310
Springfield, VA 22151
(703) 865-7162

William Sjostrom
The University of Arizona
James E. Rogers
College of Law
P.O. Box 210176
Tucson, AZ 85721
(520) 626-6451
sjostrom@email.arizona.edu

Justin Skidmore
Partner's Group
1200 Entrepreneurial Dr
Broomfield, CO 80021-8387
(303) 606-3706

Jeff Snyder
Crowell & Moring
1001 Pennsylvania Ave NW
Washington, DC 20004-2595
(202) 624-2790
jsnyder@crowell.com

John Sotirakis
Coritsidis Sotirakis & Saketos
25-61 Steinway St
Astoria, NY 11103-3739
(718) 204-0437

R. Ben Sperry
International Center
for Law & Economics
1104 NW 15th Ave
Suite 300
Portland, OR 97209
bsperry@laweconcenter.org

Mike Sporer
Sporer Mah & Co.
Tri-City Business Centre
#2300-2850 Shaughnessy St
Port Coquitlam, BC V3C 6K5
Canada
(604) 717-5510
msporer@sporermah.com

W. Randall Stroud
Araneda & Stroud
Immigration Law Group
5400 Glenwood Ave
Suite 200
Raleigh, NC 27612
(919) 788-9225
newclient@aranedalaw.com

Brandon Thibodeaux
Frilot
1100 Poydras Street
Suite 3700
New Orleans, LA 70163
(504) 599-8253
btjibodeaux@frilot.com

Maurice Thompson
Center for Constitutional Law
1851 Center
for Constitutional Law
122 E Main St
Columbus, OH 43215-4366
(614) 340-9817
mthompson
@ohioconstitution.org

Patrick Tinsley
Fletcher Tilton
1597 Falmouth Road
Centerville, MA 02632
(508) 459-8003
mansurlaw@aol.com

Maria Topakitzian
Helioupolis Law Firm
(210) 995-2020
dikeilaw@gmail.com

Fred Tung
Boston University
School of Law
765 Commonwealth Ave
Boston, MA 02215-1401
(617) 358-6184
fredtung@bu.edu

Jonathan Turley
George Washington
University
2000 H Street NW
Washington, DC 20052
(202) 994-7001
jturley@law.gwu.edu

Frank van Dun
Frank.vanDun@UGent.be

Jim Viator
Loyola University
New Orleans
College of Law
7214 St Charles Ave
Campus Box 901
New Orleans, LA 70118
jeviator@loyno.edu

Marc Victor
Attorneys for Freedom
Law Firm
3185 S. Price Rd
Chandler, AZ
(480) 755-7110
Marc@Attorneys
ForFreedom.com

Edwin Vieira Jr
13877 Napa Dr
Manassas, VA 22112
(703) 791-6780

Eugene Volokh
University of California
385 Charles E. Young Dr. East
Los Angeles, CA 90095
(310) 206-3926
volokh@law.ucla.edu

Roy Whitehead
Maricopa County
Superior Court
18380 N 40th St
Phoenix, AZ 85032-001
(602) 372-8496

B. Dean Wilson
LiMandri & Jonna, LLP
P.O. Box 9120
Rancho Santa Fe, CA 92067
(858) 759-9930
Wilsondwilson@limandri.com

Patrick Wood
pwood@revelationgate.com

Joshua Wright
Antonin Scaila Law School
George Mason University
3301 Fairfax Dr
Arlington, VA 22201
(703) 993-8236
jwrightg@gmu.edu

Todd Zywicki
George Mason University
3301 Fairfax Drive
Arlington, VA 22201
(703) 993-9484
tzywick2@gmu.edu

Acknowledgements

This book has been a community effort. The greatest online gathering of writers, readers, free men, and activists takes place each day at *LewRockwell.com*. For this, I am in debt to Mr. Rockwell, who has housed that bold community and given me a place to write for better than a decade.

Without Ron Paul, there is no freedom movement, as we today know it. On December 7, 2007, he became the grandfather of the Tea Party movement when his supporters from Strasbourg, France to Lake Jackson, Texas organized the first events in the contemporary Tea Party movement. No longer in office, this astute watchdog of government overreach and philosopher, on Tuesday, March 17, 2020, the first day of the San Francisco lockdown penned the syndicated column "The Coronavirus Hoax," in which he predicts correctly that some will die of corona, so the vulnerable must protect themselves, and that all must remain alert to the authoritarians making Covid an excuse for massive power grabs.

Gary Barnett brought passion. Becky Akers brought standards - from government, to libertarians, to God's servants on earth, boy was Becky Akers disappointed. When push came to shove, she watched the biggest talkers out there melt into the most compliant on the proving grounds of 2020. She brought friendship to that community as she blogged and reblogged the letters from the trenches.

Pastor Rich Little brought the same and a voice of mainstream Christian wisdom alongside denunciations of his tyrant governor in Michigan. From Bill Sardi to Jon Rappaport, hundreds and thousands of others magnified each other's efforts in a synergy elsewhere unmatched. Truth distilled.

The spirit of the Gadfly Majestic is a most wonderful thing to come out of 2020. It has been a gift to live through this year and to be challenged in the way this year has brought challenge. Thousands, too numerous to mention here have brought me untold inspiration by merely being their own free selves and refusing anything but that high standard in life. Though these pages do not allow the space for it, I hope to one day write at length about more of those contributions that the captive media refuses to cover.

The free man of 2020 would be the Time Man of the Year in a freer society. That is not the society in which we live, but the remnant thrives strong on the right and somewhat on the left through 2020. Any journalist with a dogged determination for the truth from Glenn Greenwald and Matt Taibbi to many others across the spectrum, are writing about the free man and critical of the predictably corrupt writing of our era. In people like that, a torch of decency is kept alive across the political spectrum. It is joy to walk the earth with such powerful souls such as these mentioned here and the Gadfly Majestic and to see them so magnificently shine against the dismal backdrop of this era. It is not the backdrop that deserves our attention, with people like this walking the earth.

For the third time in this work, I will quote a pope "Let us thank God that He makes us live among the present problems. It is no longer permitted to anyone to be mediocre." Each day I see the most magnificent examples of human inspiration.

I'm thankful to Tim Scherer, Hector Carmona, Levi & Annette Honaywax, Peter Harrigan, Steven Hertzberg, Anthony Koz, Richard Miletic, Elma Lindsay, Zack Van Wagoner, Jason T. Reynolds, Julia Pekkala, Lord Timothy McGovern, Peggy Paul, Stanley Swartzentruber, Gary Leland, Michael Hanks, Timothy Engler, Michael McEvoy, Edward Downing Jr., Kevin Young, Scott Mise, Gaynell Riley, Lee Fernandez, George Joulak, Geoff Brown, Michael James, Jeshua Richard, Gabrielle Soloma de Cadavid, Julie Pacheco, and Engin Can for their demonstrations of courage.

Nick Spanos, Stephen Qwan, Felix Brownstone, Alejandro Pasternak, Walter Block, Robert Wright for introductions and encouragement. Kate Dalley of *The Kate Dalley Show* and Tim Brown of *The Washington Standard*, Ryan McMaken of *The Mises Institute*, Joe Jarvis of *The Daily Bell*, Michael Boldin and Michael Maharrey of *The Tenth Amendment Center*, Kit Knightly of *Off Guardian*, Daniel Ivandjiiski of *Zero Hedge*, Valentin Schmid and Adam Ainsworth of *Epoch Times* for providing additional venues for these ideas.

Many thousands resisted and sent in their notes. Notes that were an inspiration to read. Notes from the corona resistance came in from all corners of the world. Among them from:

Robert E. Wright, Bo Andersen, Hoseyn Vosouq, Jeff Berwick, Kellie Hill, Mark Abell, Marc Scott, Pam Buttram, Sharine Borslien, Tazio Zatori, Jose Douglas, Ray Greninger, John Tieber, Geoffrey McKinney, Joyce Smith, Krishna Chandrasekaran, Jean Hodge, Michael F. Denny, Keith Hudson, Karen Stansberry, Elin Carlson, Alex Morris, Ashkan Jafarpisheh, Scott M. Olmsted, Vafa Faez, Judith Sanders, Gerry D. Lebow, Michelle Rice, Anthony Kujawa, Mike Maloney, Pat Goltz, Walter E. Block, Steve Swenson, Mark Higdon, Jim Sheehan, John T. Morzenti, Dave Heng, Larry Moore, David Hathaway, Bruce Bolock, Jeri Dietz, Justin Ptak, John McClain, Thomas Hyland, Walter Dubyna, Becky Akers, Ernest Roberts, Steven Ferry, Kathy Terry, John Howard, William Lensmire, Pat Palmer, Allen Nightingale, Zac Wendroff, Sam Wolanyk, Mary Beth Kaplan, Genevieve Amy Hawkins, Susan Fassanella, Ludvik Kouril, Alex Edwards, Jack Worthington, Bill Spitz, Mark Bombardier, Edward Konecnik, Mark Beck, Mike Falls, Doug Schurman, Ira Katz, Raul De La Garza III, Richard Feibel, Stephen J. Savoie, John Reilly, Charlie Beaird and DeMar Southard.

Appreciation for an additional show of inspiration is owed to Maureen Block, Alix Mayer, Robert F. Kennedy, Jr., Josh Donaldson, J.K. Monagle, Elson Haas, and Simone Gold.

These materials, alongside other work, were composed and assembled as a writer in residence at The Sonoma Harbor, Sonoma County, California, Jack London Lodge, Glen Elyn, California, Sandpiper, Carmel, California, Hotel Petaluma, Petaluma, California, Surety Stayward, Lompoc, California, Sands Inn, San Luis Obispo, California, Hill House, Mendocino County, California, and The Beach House, Mendocino County, California.

Thank you to the many people otherwise involved in this process, such as Louise Taylor, Xhudit Keli, Olha Krasikova, Muhammad Ammar, Hoorria Fatima, Adrian Gombos, Tony Weeler, Lisa Jackson, Rebecca Raouda-Saviolli, Atiar Rahman, Ryan Biore, and classicist Mia Forbes. Your efforts have been fantastic thank you. I am most appreciative to Lenka Chabalova.

My family brought drive, inspiration, and focus by being the people for whom I most wanted to be able to understand this topic and provide leadership. Their generosity and love reminded me how well successful families are able to function, even through times of crisis, or perhaps, especially through times of crisis.

Works Cited

Akers, B. (2020). Oh, Glorious Promise: "We Will Be Violating the Judge's Order"!!!!. Retrieved from https://www.lewrock well.com/lrc-blog/oh-glorious-promise-we-will-be-violating-the-judges-order/

Authors of AP News. (2020). Police: Driver wearing medical mask passed out, crashed. *AP News*. Retrieved from https://apnews.com/article/63356de8531f04d6caff2a8c90c2b 1fb

Bentley, James. (1984). *Martin Niemöller: 1892–1984*. NY: Macmillan Free Press.

Berkowitz, E. (2017). George Bush and the Americans with Disabilities Act. *Social Welfare History Project*. Retrieved from http://socialwelfare.library.vcu.edu/recollections/george-bush-and-the-americans-with-disabilities-act/

Board of Governors of the Federal Reserve System. (n.d.). What is the purpose of the Federal Reserve System?. Retrieved from https://www.federalreserve.gov/faqs/about_ 12594.html

Brantley, K. (2020). New Jersey driver wearing an N95 mask for hours crashes after passing out behind the wheel from lack of oxygen. *The Daily Mail*. Retrieved from https://www.daily mail.co.uk/news/article-8256631/New-Jersey-driver-wearing-N95-mask-hours-crashes-passing-out.html

Carlin, G. (2017). George Carlin: Doin' It Again (1990)- Transcript. Retrieved from https://scrapsfromtheloft.com/2017/06/27/george-carlin-doin-1990-transcript/

Carnegie, Andrew. (1889). The Best Fields for Philanthropy. *North American Review*. 149: 688– 691.

Carrega, C. (2020). Driver in crash may have passed out from wearing N95 mask too long: Police. *ABC News*. Retrieved from https://abcnews.go.com/US/driver-crash-passed-wearing-n95-mask-long-police/story?id=70346532

Centres for Disease Control and Prevention. (1996). Health Insurance Portability and Accountability Act of 1996 (HIPAA). Retrieved from https://www.cdc.gov/phlp/publications/topic/hipaa.html

Centres for Disease Control and Prevention. (2020). Considerations for Wearing Masks. Retrieved from https://www.cdc.gov/coronavirus/2019-ncov/prevent-getting-sick/cloth-face-cover-guidance.html

Centres for Disease Control and Prevention. (2020). Coronavirus Disease 2019 (COVID-19): Know How It Spreads. Retrieved from https:/www.cdc.gov/coronavirus/2019-ncov/prevent-getting-sick/prevention.html

Centres for Disease Control and Prevention. (2020). JAMA editorial reviews latest science, while case study shows masks prevented COVID spread. Retrieved from https://www.cdc.gov/media/releases/2020/p0714-americans-to-wear-masks.html

Centres for Disease Control and Prevention. (2020). Staff. Retrieved from https://wwwnc.cdc.gov/eid/about/staff

Chammah, M. (2020). The Rise of the Anti-Lockdown Sheriffs. *The Marshall Project*. Retrieved from https://www.themarshallproject.org/2020/05/18/the-rise-of-the-anti-lockdown-sheriffs

Chen, S. (2008). How to play the first bar of Rhapsody in Blue. *The Journal of the Acoustical Society of America*, *123*(5), 3123–3123. Retrieved from https://doi.org/10.1121.1.2933048

Clear, J. (n.d.). Rome Wasn't Built in a Day, But They Were Laying Bricks Every Hour. Retrieved from https://jamesclear.com/lay-a-brick

Collman, A. (2020). An Orthodox Jewish community in Brooklyn burned face masks in a bonfire to protest Gov. Cuomo imposing a local coronavirus lockdown on them *Business Insider*. Retrieved from https://www.businessinsider.com/nyc-orthodox-jews-protest-local-lockdown-face-masks-bonfire-2020-10

Contrera, J. (2020). The N95 shortage America can't seem to fix. *The Washington Post*. Retrieved from https://www.washingtonpost.com/graphics/2020/local/news/n-95-shortage-covid/

Crespolini, R., Patch Staff. (2020). N95 Mask-Wearing Morris Co. Driver Passes Out, Crashes Car: Cops. *Patch*. Retrieved from https://patch.com/new-jersey/parsippany/n95-mask-wearing-nj-driver-passes-out-crashes-car-police

Danner, C. (2020). Philly Police Drag Man From Bus for Not Wearing a Face Mask. *New York Magazine*. Retrieved from https://nymag.com/intelligencer/2020/04/philly-police-drag-man-from-bus-for-not-wearing-a-face-mask.html

Dehlendorf, C., Harris, L. H., & Weitz, T. A. (2013). Disparities in abortion rates: a public health approach. *American journal of public health*, *103*(10), 1772–1779. Retrieved from https://doi.org/10.2105/AJPH.2013.301339

Deibert, B. (2019). What is the Golden Rule?- Biblical Meaning, Importance and Examples. Retrieved from https://www.christianity.com/christian-life/what-is-the-golden-rule.html

Delta Airlines. (n.d.). Travelers with Disabilities. Retrieved from https://pro.delta.com/content/agency/us/en/products-and-services/special-services/travelerswith- disabilities.html#

Deviva, J.C., & Zayfert, C. (2011). *When Someone You Love Suffers from Posttraumatic Stress: What to Expect and What You Can Do (1st Edition)*. The Guilford Press.

Exec. Order No. 2020-153: Masks, *rescission of* Exec. Order No. 2020-147 (2020). Retrieved from https://www.michigan.gov/whitmer/0,9309,7-387-90499_90705-535105--,00.html

Ferguson, N.M., Laydon, D., Nedjati-Gilani, G., Imai, N., Ainslie, K., Baguelin, M.,...Ghani, A.C. (2020). Report 9: Impact of non-pharmaceutical interventions (NPIs) to reduce COVID-19 mortality and healthcare demand. *Imperial College COVID-19 Response Team*. Retrieved from https://www.imperial.ac.uk/media/imperial-college/medicine/sph/ide/gida-fellowships/Imperial-College-COVID19-NPI-modelling-16-03-2020.pdf

Fong, G. (2020). Nonpharmaceutical Measures for Pandemic Influenza in Nonhealthcare Settings—Social Distancing Measures. *Emerging Infectious Diseases, 26*(5), 976–984. Retrieved from https://doi.org/10.3201/eid2605.190995

Frail, T.A. (2017). The Injustice of Japanese-American Internment Camps Resonates Strongly to This Day. *Smithsonian Magazine*. Retrieved from https://www.smithsonianmag.com/history/injustice-japanese-americans-internment-camps-resonates-strongly-180961422/

Gomez, J. (2020). Lincoln Park driver 'passed out' due to N95 mask, crashed car, police say. *Morristown Daily Record*. Retrieved from https://www.dailyrecord.com/story/news/2020/04/24/lincoln-park-driver-passed-out-due-n-95-mask-crashed-car-police-said/3021288001/

Hanau, S. (2020). Orthodox Jews in Brooklyn burn masks during massive protest against New York's new COVID rules. Jewish Telegraphic Agency. Retrieved from https://www.jta.org/2020/10/07/health/orthodox-jews-in-brooklyn-burn-masks-during-massive-protest-against-new-yorks-new-covid-restrictions

Haywood, B. (2010). 2010 Construction Accidents. Retrieved from https://www.safteng.net/index.php/33-incident-alert-archives/construction-accidents

History.com Editors. (2009). President Eisenhower warns of military-industrial complex. Retrieved from https://www.history.com/this-day-in-history/eisenhower-warns-of-military-industrial-complex

History.com Editors. (2010). League of Nations Instituted. Retrieved from https://www.history.com/this-day-in-history/league-of-nations-instituted

History.com Editors. (2019). Armenian Genocide. Retrieved from https://www.history.com/topics/world-war-i/armenian-genocide

Holt, A. (2017). 100 Million Victims of Communism. Retrieved from https://apholt.com/2017/07/02/100-million-victims-of-communism/

Holt, A. (2018). The 20th century's Bloodiest "Megamurderers" according to Prof. R.J. Rummel. Retrieved from https://apholt.com/2018/11/15/the-20th-centurys-bloodiest-megamurderers-according-to-prof-r-j-rummel/

Johnson A. T. (2016). Respirator masks protect health but impact performance: a review. *Journal of biological engineering*, *10*, 4. Retrieved from https://doi.org/10.1186/s13036-016-0025-4

Kornfield, M. (2020). Three people charged in killing of Family Dollar security over mask policy. *The Washington Post*. Retrieved from https://www.washingtonpost.com/nation/2020/05/04/security-guards-death-might-have-been-because-he-wouldnt-let-woman-store-without-mask

Macias, T. (2020). Man without face mask turns violent when he's asked to leave Texas store, video shows. *Fort Worth Star-Telegram*. Retrieved from https://www.star-telegram.com/news/coronavirus/article242761841.html

Maine Department of Economic & Community Development. (2020). Covid-19 Prevention Checklists. Retrieved from https://www.maine.gov/decd/covid-19-prevention-checklists

Mascia, J. (2020). People Keep Shooting Each Other Over Coronavirus Restrictions. *The Trace*. Retrieved from https://www.thetrace.org/2020/05/coronavirus-restrictions-social-distancing-shootings-tracker

Mase, S.R. (2020). Order of the Health Officer C19-07: Facial Coverings. *SoCo Emergency- County of Sonoma California*. Retrieved from https://socoemergency.org/order-of-the-health-officer-facial-coverings/

Matsakis, A.T. (2014). *Loving Someone with PTSD: A Practical Guide to Understanding and Connecting with Your Partner after Trauma (The New Harbinger Loving Someone Series)* (1st Edition). New Harbinger Publications.

McCarthy, C. (2020). New Jersey driver crashes car after passing out from wearing N95 mask. *New York Post*. Retrieved from https://nypost.com/2020/04/24/driver-crashes-car-after-passing-out-from-wearing-n95-mask/

McKeever, A. (2020). How the Americans with Disabilities Act transformed a country. *National Geographic*. Retrieved from https://www.nationalgeographic.com/history/2020/07/americans-disabilities-act-transformed-united-states/

Menger, C., Hayek, F.A., Klein, P.G., Dingwall, J., Hoselitz, B.F. (2007). *Principles of Economics*. Auburn, AL: Ludwig von Mises Institute.

National Institute of Mental Health. (2017). Panic Disorder. Retrieved from https://www.nimh.nih.gov/health/statistics/panic-disorder.shtml

Oil Sands Magazine. (2017). WTI Specs Get a Minor Makeover in 2018. Retrieved from https://www.oilsandsmagazine.com/news/2017/12/22/west-texas-intermediate-wti-specifications-get-updated-in-2018

Oral Health. (2016). Update: Why Face Masks Don't Work: A Revealing Review. Retrieved from https://www.oralhealthgroup.com/features/face-masks-dont-work-revealing-review/

Patray, B. (2019). More Black Babies in New York City are Killed in Abortions Than Born Alive. *Tennessee Eagle Forum*. Retrieved from http://tneagleforum.org/blog_direct_link.cfm?blog_id=65521

Riley, J.L. (2018). Let's Talk About the Black Abortion Rate. *The Wall Street Journal*. Retrieved from https://www.wsj.com/articles/lets-talk-about-the-black-abortion-rate-1531263697

Roberge, R. J., Coca, A., Williams, W. J., Powell, J. B., & Palmiero, A. J. (2010). Physiological impact of the N95 filtering facepiece respirator on healthcare workers. *Respiratory care*, *55*(5), 569–577.

Roberge, R. J., Coca, A., Williams, W. J., Powell, J. B., & Palmiero, A. J. (2010). Physiological impact of the N95 filtering facepiece respirator on healthcare workers. *Respiratory care*, *55*(5), 569–577.

Romeo, J. (2020). Altercation over face masks escalates into violence at Durango store. *The Durango Herald*. Retrieved from https://durangoherald.com/articles/334940

Rummel, R. (1994). *Death by Government*. Transaction Publishers.

Sacramento Metropolitan Fire, Sacramento County Department of Health Services Public Health Division. (2018). *N95 Respirator Announcement*. Retrieved from https://www.metro fire.ca.gov/index.php/news-releases/889-n95-respirator-announcement

Satter, D. (2017). 100 Years of Communism—and 100 Million Dead. *Hudson Institute*. Retrieved from https://www.hud son.org/research/13994-100-years-of-communism-and-100-million-dead

Sawers, P. (2020). Brave browser taps the Wayback Machine to show deleted web pages. *Venture Beat*. Retrieved from https://venturebeat.com/2020/02/26/brave-browser-taps-the-wayback-machine-to-show-deleted-web-pages/

Seiger, T. (2020). Man shot, killed by deputy after fight over wearing mask, reports say. *Fox23 News*. Retrieved from https://www.fox23.com/news/trending/man-shot-killed-by-police-after-fight-over-wearing-mask-reports-say/CE6ORWE6UVBBPGOLCZZTREBRQI/

Shakespeare, W. (2013). Henry V. CreateSpace Independent Publishing Platform. (Original Work published 1599)

Slings, S.R. (1994). *Plato's Apology of Socrates: A Literary and Philosophical Study with a Running Commentary*. E.J. Brill.

Spectator, H. (2020). Grocery store fight over masks turns violent in Tillsonburg. *HamiltonNews.com*. Retrieved from https://www.hamiltonnews.com/news-story/9986576-grocery-store-fight-over-masks-turns-violent-

Stack, L. (2020). Backlash Grows in Orthodox Jewish Areas Over Virus Crackdown by Cuomo. T*he New York Times*. Retrieved from https://www.nytimes.com/2020/10/07/nyregion/orthodox-jews-nyc-coronavirus.html

Stevo, A.J. (2015). In Poems. *CreateSpace Independent Publishing Platform*.

Telford, Taylor. (2020). Marriott, the world's largest hotel chain, will require guests to wear masks in common areas. *The Washington Post*. Retrieved from https://www.washingtonpost.com/travel/2020/07/21/marriott-worlds-largest-hotel-chain-will-require-guests-wear-masks-common-areas/

Texas Public Law. (2019). Texas Education Code-Sec. 37.0023 Prohibited Averisve Techniques. Retrieved from https://texas.public.law/statutes/tex._educ._code_section_37.0023

U.S. Department of Education. (n.d.). Grant Application and Other Forms. Retrieved from https://www2.ed.gov/fund/grant/apply/appforms/appforms.html

United Nations. (n.d.). History of the United Nations. Retrieved from https://www.un.org/en/sections/history/history-united-nations/index.html

VanSlyck, A.A. (1991). The Utmost Amount of Effectiv [sic] Accommodation: Andrew Carnegie and the Reform of the American Library. *Journal of the Society of Architectural Historians*. 50 (4): 359–83.

Washington's Blog. (2019). America Has Been at War 93% of the Time – 222 out of 239 Years – Since 1776. *Global Research*. Retrieved from https://www.globalresearch.ca/america-has-been-at-war-93-of-the-time-222-out-of-239-years-since-1776/5565946

Webb, K. (2020). Man arrested after pulling gun during mask argument at Florida Walmart. *USA Today.* Retrieved from https://www.usatoday.com/story/news/nation/2020/07/24/ma n-arrested-after-pulling-gun-mask-argument-florida-walmart/5501266002/

West Virgina Sports. (2020). How To Sue Your Governor... . Retrieved from https://westvirginia.forums.rivals.com/threads/ how-to-sue-your-governor.229564/

Williamson County Liberitarian Party. (n.d.). You May Be Exempt From Wearing a Face Mask. Retrieved from https://txwclp.org/2020/05/you-may-be-exempt-from-wearing-a-face-mask/

Wilson, J. (2020). US sheriffs rebel against state mask orders even as Covid-19 spreads. *The Guardian.* Retrieved from https://www.theguardian.com/us-news/2020/jul/31/us-sheriffs-mask-orders-covid-19-blm

Woodward, A. (2020). Driver crashes after passing out from 'excessive wearing' of coronavirus face mask. *Independent.* Retrieved from https://www.independent.co.uk/news/world/ americas/car-crash-new-jersey-face-mask-new-jersey-lincoln-park-police-a9484236.html

World Health Organization. (2009). Advice on the use of masks1 in the community setting in Influenza A (H1N1) out-breaks. Retrieved from https://www.who.int/csr/resources/ publications/Adviceusemaskscommunityrevised.pdf

Wright, R.E., (2020). Why Aren't Americans Suing Their Way Out of Lockdown?. American Institute for Economic Research. Retrieved from https://www.aier.org/article/why-arent-ameri cans-suing-their-way-out-of-lockdown/

Xiao, J., Shiu, E., Gao, H., Wong, J. Y., Fong, M. W., Ryu, S....Cowling, B. J. (2020). Nonpharmaceutical Measures for Pandemic Influenza in Nonhealthcare Settings—Personal Protective and Environmental Measures. *Emerging Infectious Diseases, 26*(5), 967-975. Retrieved from https://dx.doi.org/ 10.3201/eid2605.190994.

Yolo County. (n.d.). Unhealthy Air Quality Guidance. Retrieved from https://www.yolocounty.org/health-human-services/health-alerts/unhealthy-air-quality-guidance

Endnotes

[1] Xiao, J., Shiu, E., Gao, H., Wong, J. Y., Fong, M. W., Ryu, S....Cowling, B. J. (2020). Nonpharmaceutical Measures for Pandemic Influenza in Nonhealthcare Settings—Personal Protective and Environmental Measures. *Emerging Infectious*

[2] Bob Barker - Bob Barker was an entertainer in the late 20th and early 21st century who hosted a game show called "The Price is Right," in which contestants could win cars, vacations, and other prices.

[3] Andrew Carnegie - Andrew Carnegie was a successful businessman of the late 19th and early 20th century who used his wealth partly to gift libraries. Carnegie is believed to have gifted some 3,000 libraries to communities, largely in the United States, but also around the world.
VanSlyck, A.A. (1991). The Utmost Amount of Effectiv [sic] Accommodation: Andrew Carnegie and the Reform of the American Library. *Journal of the Society of Architectural Historians.* 50 (4): 359–83.
As Van Slyck (1991) showed, during the last years of the 19th century, there was increasing adoption of the idea that free libraries should be available to the American public. But the design of such libraries was the subject of prolonged and heated debate. On one hand, the library profession called for designs that supported efficiency in administration and operation; on the other, wealthy philanthropists favored buildings that reinforced the paternalistic metaphor and enhanced civic pride. Between 1886 and 1917, Carnegie reformed both library philanthropy and library design, encouraging a closer correspondence between the two.

[4] Carnegie, Andrew. (1889). The Best Fields for Philanthropy. *North American Review.* 149: 688– 691.
A Carnegie library is a library built with money donated by Scottish-American businessman and philanthropist Andrew Carnegie. A total of 2,509 Carnegie libraries were built between 1883 and 1929, including some belonging to public and university library systems. 1,689 were built in the United States, 660 in the United Kingdom and Ireland, 125 in Canada, and others in Australia, South Africa, New Zealand, Serbia, Belgium, France, the Caribbean, Mauritius, Malaysia, and Fiji. At first, Carnegie libraries were almost exclusively in places with which he had a personal connection — namely his birthplace in Scotland and the Pittsburgh, Pennsylvania area, his adopted home-town. Yet, beginning in the middle of 1899, Carnegie substantially increased funding to libraries outside these areas. In later years few towns that requested a grant and agreed to his terms, of committing to operation and maintenance, were refused. By the time the last grant was made in 1919, there were 3,500 libraries in the United States, nearly half of them known as Carnegie libraries, as they were built with construction grants paid by Carnegie. Nearly all of Carnegie's libraries were built according to "the Carnegie formula," which required financial commitments for maintenance and operation from the town that received the donation. Carnegie required public support rather than making endowments because, as he wrote: "an endowed institution is liable to become the prey of a clique. The public ceases to take interest in it, or, rather, never acquires interest in it. The rule has

been violated which requires the recipients to help themselves. Everything has been done for the community instead of its being only helped to help itself."

Carnegie required the elected officials—the local government—to: demonstrate the need for a public library; provide the building site; pay staff and maintain the library; draw from public funds to run the library—not use only private donations; annually provide ten percent of the cost of the library's construction to support its operation; and, provide free service to all.

[5] Ad nauseam - Nausea comes from the Greek for "sea" and is accordingly the condition of being on the sea, or "sea-sickness," as it is commonly called in this era in English. Nausea has been generalized to mean a feeling of sickness or unease with an inclination to vomit. There are plenty of behaviors to which people have a physical revulsion, and which their bodies are telling them not to engage: the wrong work, deceit, bad decisions, or talking to people you don't care for could all be examples. This is an era in which many are encouraged to do things that make them nauseous so frequently that they grow immune to the sense of nausea. Nausea is a protective sense that says "Stop. Get away from this. Examine the situation from a distance." Little wisdom of that kind is able to be gleaned in this era. To ignore instinct is the prevailing suggestion of the era. As such the term ad nauseam has lost considerable meaning. It is practically considered heroic in this era to entirely ignore instinct, while what was once called heroism has been redefined with all manner of pejoratives.

[6] Clear, J. (n.d.). Rome Wasn't Built in a Day, But They Were Laying Bricks Every Hour. Retrieved from https://jamesclear.com/lay-a-brick
James Clear writes "John Heywood was an English playwright who lived hundreds of years ago. Today, Heywood is known for his poems, proverbs, and plays. But more than any one work, it's his phrases that have made him famous. For example, here are some popular sayings that have been attributed to Heywood... 'Out of sight out of mind.' 'Better late than never.' 'The more the merrier.' 'Many hands make light work.' And there is one phrase from Heywood that is particularly interesting when it comes to building better habits: 'Rome was not built in one day.'"

[7] Wilson, J. (2020). US sheriffs rebel against state mask orders even as Covid-19 spreads. *The Guardian*. Retrieved from https://www.theguardian.com/us-news/2020/jul/31/us-sheriffs-mask-orders-covid-19-blm

[8] Chammah, M. (2020). The Rise of the Anti-Lockdown Sheriffs. *The Marshall Project*. Retrieved from https://www.themarshallproject.org/2020/05/18/the-rise-of-the-anti-lockdown-sheriffs
Examples of sheriffs who have taken courageous public stands on this matter include: Sheriff Adam Fortney, in Snohomish County, Washington; Chad Bianco, the sheriff of Riverside County, California; Herrington, sheriff of Chaves County, New Mexico; Sheriff Daryl Wheeler, Idaho; Sheriff Christopher Schmaling, Racine County, Wisconsin; Sheriff Scott Nichols, Franklin County, Maine; Richard K Jones, Sheriff of Butler County, Ohio; Tracy Murphee, Denton County Sheriff, Texas; Jimmy Thorton, Sampson County Sheriff, North Carolina Rob Snaza, Lewis County Sheriff, Washington.

[9] Quietly – If you have enough conversations with police about face masks the number of them will have no faith on this topic they are being asked to enforce is enormous. They tend to be very realistic about such hysterics because they recognize the unenforceable nature of a law will cause the law to be null regardless how passionately some lawmakers thinks it's a great idea. Reality may simply have a different agenda. This reality gives rise to the statement "man proposes, God disposes," or "man plans, good laughs."

[10] Mase, S.R. (2020). Order of the Health Officer C19-07: Facial Coverings. *SoCo Emergency- County of Sonoma California*. Retrieved from https://socoemergen cy.org/order-of-the-health-officer-facial-coverings/

[11] Exec. Order No. 2020-153: Masks, *rescission of* Exec. Order No. 2020-147 (2020). Retrieved from https://www.michigan.gov/whitmer/0,9309,7-387-90499_ 90705-535105--,00.html

[12] Deibert, B. (2019). What is the Golden Rule?- Biblical Meaning, Importance and Examples. Retrieved from https://www.christianity.com/christian-life/what-is-the-golden-rule.html
Golden Rule - The Golden Rule is the ethical principle of treating other people as one's self would prefer to be treated. One of Jesus' most famous and impactful teachings, the Golden Rule can be found in the Bible verses Matthew 7:12 and Luke 6:31: "So in everything, do to others what you would have them do to you, for this sums up the Law and the Prophets." Matthew 7:12 "Do to others as you would have them do to you." Luke 6:31

[13] Yolo County. (n.d.). Unhealthy Air Quality Guidance. Retrieved from https://www.yolocounty.org/health-human-services/health-alerts/unhealthy-air-quality-guidance

[14] Sacramento Metropolitan Fire, Sacramento County Department of Health Services Public Health Division. (2018). *N95 Respirator Announcement*. Retrieved from https://www.metrofire.ca.gov/index.php/news-releases/889-n95-respirator-announcement

[15] Johnson A. T. (2016). Respirator masks protect health but impact performance: a review. *Journal of biological engineering*, *10*, 4. Retrieved from https://doi.org/10.1186/s13036-016-0025-4

[16] Roberge, R. J., Coca, A., Williams, W. J., Powell, J. B., & Palmiero, A. J. (2010). Physiological impact of the N95 filtering facepiece respirator on healthcare workers. *Respiratory care*, *55*(5), 569–577.

[17] Roberge, R. J., Coca, A., Williams, W. J., Powell, J. B., & Palmiero, A. J. (2010). Physiological impact of the N95 filtering facepiece respirator on healthcare workers. Respiratory care, 55(5), 569–577.

[18] Carrega, C. (2020). Driver in crash may have passed out from wearing N95 mask too long: Police. *ABC News*. Retrieved from https://abcnews.go.com/US/driver-crash-passed-wearing-n95-mask-long-police/story?id=70346532

[19] Gomez, J. (2020). Lincoln Park driver 'passed out' due to N95 mask, crashed car, police say. *Morristown Daily Record*. Retrieved from https://www.dailyrecord.com/story/news/2020/04/24/lincoln-park-driver-passed-out-due-n-95-mask-crashed-car-police-said/3021288001/

[20] McCarthy, C. (2020). New Jersey driver crashes car after passing out from wearing N95 mask. *New York Post*. Retrieved from https://nypost.com/2020/04/24/driver-crashes-car-after-passing-out-from-wearing-n95-mask/

[21] Authors of AP News. (2020). Police: Driver wearing medical mask passed out, crashed. *AP News*. Retrieved from https://apnews.com/article/63356de8531f04d6caff2a8c90c2b1fb

[22] Woodward, A. (2020). Driver crashes after passing out from 'excessive wearing' of coronavirus face mask. *Independent*. Retrieved from https://www.independent.co.uk/news/world/americas/car-crash-new-jersey-face-mask-new-jersey-lincoln-park-police-a9484236.html

[23] Crespolini, R., Patch Staff. (2020). N95 Mask-Wearing Morris Co. Driver Passes Out, Crashes Car: Cops. *Patch*. Retrieved from https://patch.com/new-jersey/parsippany/n95-mask-wearing-nj-driver-passes-out-crashes-car-police

[24] Brantley, K. (2020). New Jersey driver wearing an N95 mask for hours crashes after passing out behind the wheel from lack of oxygen. *The Daily Mail*. Retrieved from https://www.dailymail.co.uk/news/article-8256631/New-Jersey-driver-wearing-N95-mask-hours-crashes-passing-out.html

[25] Contrera, J. (2020). The N95 shortage America can't seem to fix. *The Washington Post*. Retrieved from https://www.washingtonpost.com/graphics/2020/local/news/n-95-shortage-covid/

[26] Haywood, B. (2010). 2010 Construction Accidents. Retrieved from https://www.safteng.net/index.php/33-incident-alert-archives/construction-accidents

[27] Williamson County Libertarian Party. (n.d.). You May Be Exempt From Wearing a Face Mask. Retrieved from https://txwclp.org/2020/05/you-may-be-exempt-from-wearing-a-face-mask/

[28] Oral Health. (2016). Update: Why Face Masks Don't Work: A Revealing Review. Retrieved from https://www.oralhealthgroup.com/features/face-masks-dont-work-revealing-review/

29 Oral Health. (2016). Update: Why Face Masks Don't Work: A Revealing Review. Retrieved from https://www.oralhealthgroup.com/features/face-masks-dont-work-revealing-review/

30 Blumberg, J. (2007). A Brief History of the Salem Witch Trials. The Smithsonian Magazine. Retrieved from https://www.smithsonianmag.com/history/a-brief-history-of-the-salem-witch-trials-175162489/

31 An axiom is a statement regarded as self-evidently true. Great work is undertaken to discover the truth. Not everyone does that work. Not everyone who does that work walks the same path in the same order. Speaking in axioms can cause one to be severely misunderstood by those who do not know the path walked or the person speaking. It does however cut to the chase and offers distilled truth, sometimes a little too potent for the uninitiated.

32 McKeever, A. (2020). How the Americans with Disabilities Act transformed a country. *National Geographic*. Retrieved from https://www.nationalgeographic.com/history/2020/07/americans-disabilities-act-transformed-united-states/

33 Centers for Disease Control and Prevention. (1996). Health Insurance Portability and Accountability Act of 1996 (HIPAA). Retrieved from https://www.cdc.gov/phlp/publications/topic/hipaa.html

34 This fearful behavior is even more common among those referenced as front line workers. – Front line – The term front line used to mean where to opposing armies met. It was the place of greater risk, greater bravery, and greater heroics. With so few people first hand engaging in war in the English speaking world, the term front line has come to lose its meaning. Front line now means "person who I want to artificially inflate the ego, authority, or view of." It means nearly nothing else in the popular English language use of the word at this point in history.

35 3,141 American counties – It's hard to precisely measure the number of counties in the United States, though the number 3,141 is commonly cited and approximately accurate. Based on how you define county, and how you define the United States, this number has approximately a 3% margin of error. As such, this number is far more accurate than the global public health pronouncement claiming face masks slow the spread of Covid-19.

36 John Locke – John Locke is a commonly cited writer across the political spectrum. Though I am unable to specifically point to a way that made him any different from those who came before, to whom he was often enough inferior and in so many ways, I disproportionately hear his name.

331

[37] Young Turks – Named for a terrorist organization, The Young Turks were a news opinion team active in the first part of the twenty–first century in the United States with an off–kilter, quasi–professional way about them that fit the new media of the era well.
History.com Editors. (2019). Armenian Genocide. Retrieved from https://www.history.com/topics/world-war-i/armenian-genocide

[38] Twitter – Twitter is the name of a micro–blogging platform popular in the first part of the twenty–first century. It gave users the ability to share very short messages easily.

[39] Fox – Fox is an international news media and entertainment conglomerate active in the second half of the twentieth century and first part of the twenty–first century. It is popularly seen as "far right," but is as technocratic and pro-establishment as any other news source. Seldom will a topic of any consequence be dealt with in any pro-technocrat and pro-establishment news source like Fox, CNN, The New York Times, or any of the many virtually indistinguishable other news sources era. Tremendous budget markets are spent by such companies to fool viewers and advertisers alike into seeing how very different they are. Occasionally, a short-lived commentary or journalist has success breaking the mold, a success often short-lived. Either he falls in line or is encouraged to seek employment elsewhere.

[40] Menger, C., Hayek, F.A., Klein, P.G., Dingwall, J., Hoselitz, B.F. (2007). *Principles of Economics*. Auburn, AL: Ludwig von Mises Institute.

[41] Webb, K. (2020). Man arrested after pulling gun during mask argument at Florida Walmart. *USA Today*. Retrieved from https://www.usatoday.com/story/news/nation/2020/07/24/man-arrested-after-pulling-gun-mask-argument-florida-walmart/5501266002/

[42] Hutchinson, B. (2020). 'Incomprehensible': Confrontations over masks erupt amid COVID-19 crisis. ABC News. Retrieved from https://abcnews.go.com/US/incomprehensible-confrontations-masks-erupt-amid-covid-19-crisis/story?id=70494577

[43] 4. Danner, C. (2020). Philly Police Drag Man From Bus for Not Wearing a Face Mask. New York Magazine. Retrieved from https://nymag.com/intelligencer/2020/04/philly-police-drag-man-from-bus-for-not-wearing-a-face-mask.html

[44] Spectator, H. (2020). Grocery store fight over masks turns violent in Tillsonburg. *HamiltonNews.com*. Retrieved from https://www.hamiltonnews.com/news-story/9986576-grocery-store-fight-over-masks-turns-violent-

[45] Macias, T. (2020). Man without face mask turns violent when he's asked to leave Texas store, video shows. *Fort Worth Star-Telegram*. Retrieved from https://www.star-telegram.com /news/coronavirus/article242761841.html

[46] Romeo, J. (2020). Altercation over face masks escalates into violence at Durango store. *The Durango Herald*. Retrieved from https://durangoherald.com/articles/334940

[47] Mascia, J. (2020). People Keep Shooting Each Other Over Coronavirus Restrictions. *The Trace*. Retrieved from https://www.thetrace.org/2020/05/coronavirus-restrictions-social-distancing-shootings-tracker/

[48] McCollough, M. (2020). Tensions Over Masks, Social Distancing Lead To Violent Altercations, Shooting Death, Pipe Bomb Threats. Kaiser Health News. Retrieved from https://khn.org/morning-breakout/tensions-over-masks-social-distancing-lead-to-violent-altercations-shooting-death-pipe-bomb-threats/

[49] Kornfield, M. (2020). Three people charged in killing of Family Dollar security over mask policy. *The Washington Post*. Retrieved from https://www.washingtonpost.com/nation/2020/05/04/security-guards-death-might-have-been-because-he-wouldnt-let-woman-store-without-mask

[50] Seiger, T. (2020). Man shot, killed by deputy after fight over wearing mask, reports say. *Fox23 News*. Retrieved from https://www.fox23.com/news/trending/man-shot-killed-by-police-after-fight-over-wearing-mask-reports-say/CE6ORWE6UVBBPGOLCZZTREBRQI/

[51] Frail, T.A. (2017). The Injustice of Japanese-American Internment Camps Resonates Strongly to This Day. Smithsonian Magazine. Retrieved from https://www.smithsonianmag.com/history/injustice-japanese-americans-internment-camps-resonates-strongly-180961422/

[52] Satter, D. (2017). 100 Years of Communism—and 100 Million Dead. *Hudson Institute*. Retrieved from https://www.hudson.org/research/13994-100-years-of-communism-and-100-million-dead

[53] Holt, A. (2017). 100 Million Victims of Communism. Retrieved from https://apholt.com/2017/07/02/100-million-victims-of-communism/

[54] Holt, A. (2018). The 20th century's Bloodiest "Megamurderers" according to Prof. R.J. Rummel. Retrieved from https://apholt.com/2018/11/15/the-20th-centurys-bloodiest-megamurderers-according-to-prof-r-j-rummel/

[55] Rummel, R. (1994). *Death by Government*. Transaction Publishers.

[56] Riley, J.L. (2018). Let's Talk About the Black Abortion Rate. *The Wall Street Journal*. Retrieved from https://www.wsj.com/articles/lets-talk-about-the-black-abortion-rate-1531263697

[57] Riley, J.L. (2018). Let's Talk About the Black Abortion Rate. *The Wall Street Journal*. Retrieved from https://www.wsj.com/articles/lets-talk-about-the-black-abortion-rate-1531263697

[58] Center for Urban Renewal and Education. (2015). Policy Report: The Effects of Abortion on the Black Community. (Cure Document 202.479.2873). Washington, DC: U.S. House of Representatives. https://docs.house.gov/meetings/JU/JU10/20171101/106562/HHRG-115-JU10-Wstate-ParkerS-20171101-SD001.pdf

[59] Dehlendorf, C., Harris, L. H., & Weitz, T. A. (2013). Disparities in abortion rates: a public health approach. *American journal of public health*, *103*(10), 1772–1779. Retrieved from https://doi.org/10.2105/AJPH.2013.301339

[60] Patray, B. (2019). More Black Babies in New York City are Killed in Abortions Than Born Alive. *Tennessee Eagle Forum*. Retrieved from http://tneagleforum.org/blog_direct_link.cfm?blog_id=65521

[61] Washington's Blog. (2019). America Has Been at War 93% of the Time – 222 out of 239 Years – Since 1776. *Global Research*. Retrieved from https://www.globalresearch.ca/america-has-been-at-war-93-of-the-time-222-out-of-239-years-since-1776/5565946
Since the United States was founded in 1776, she has been at war during 214 out of her 235 calendar years of existence. In other words, there were only 21 calendar years in which the U.S. did not wage any wars.
To put this in perspective:
* Pick any year since 1776 and there is about a 91% chance that America was involved in some war during that calendar year.
* No U.S. president truly qualifies as a peacetime president. Instead, all U.S. presidents can technically be considered "war presidents."
* The U.S. has never gone a decade without war.
* The only time the U.S. went five years without war (1935-40) was during the isolationist period of the Great Depression.

[62] Deus ex machina - In Greek tragedy, this is he who descends from on high to help bring the play to a resolution and perhaps even "save the day." This is not a useful view of reality, to wait for someone to save the day. It is entirely contrary to all indication of reality to expect anyone in Washington DC to save the day. It is simply not something even possible to accomplish within our current system, as no solution will please all and the closest to a solution that would be possible would be agreeing to let each person pursue his own objective without interference from DC.

[63] National Institute of Mental Health. (2017). Panic Disorder. Retrieved from https://www.nimh.nih.gov/health/statistics/panic-disorder.shtml

[64] Oral Health. (2016). Update: Why Face Masks Don't Work: A Revealing Review. Retrieved from https://www.oralhealthgroup.com/features/face-masks-dont-work-revealing-review/

[65] Oral Health. (2016). Update: Why Face Masks Don't Work: A Revealing Review. Retrieved from https://www.oralhealthgroup.com/features/face-masks-dont-work-revealing-review/

[66] Sawers, P. (2020). Brave browser taps the Wayback Machine to show deleted web pages. *Venture Beat*. Retrieved from https://venturebeat.com/2020/02/26/brave-browser-taps-the-wayback-machine-to-show-deleted-web-pages/

[67] Carlin, G. (2017). George Carlin: Doin' It Again (1990)- Transcript. Retrieved from https://scrapsfromtheloft.com/2017/06/27/george-carlin-doin-1990-transcript

[68] On Thursday, August 13, 2020, Joe Biden and Kamala Harris, minor politicians of that era who temporarily had a national platform as candidates for President and Vice President respectively, appeared together at a press conference at which they called for three months of mandatory face masks orders. Biden said the following: "Every single American should be wearing a mask when they're outside for the next three months at a minimum. Every governor should mandate, every governor should mandate mandatory mask wearing. The estimates by the experts are it will save over 40,000 lives in the next three months — 40,000 lives — if people act responsibly. And it's not about your rights. It's about your responsibilities as an American. So let's institute a mask mandate, nationwide, starting immediately and we will save lives. The estimates are we'll save over 40,000 lives in the next three months if that is done." Harris said the following: "That's what real leadership looks like. We just witnessed real leadership, which is Joe Biden said that as a nation, we should all be wearing a mask for the next three months because it will save lives. And the thing about Joe that the American people know is that his role of leadership in our country has always been about doing what's best for the people of our country." Their brief, carefully crafted, prepared statements overlapped on one topic – all governors should institute face mask orders for the following three months. National elections were three months later, on November 3, 2020.

[69] Some live to tell a story. Among them are those in the media. Stories are an important part of life. To make the story the primary goal in life, or even the cause of life, promises to pervert life. Though storytellers are very valuable to a society, those who place the telling of stories as primary in their life must be well insulated and not allowed to touch the precious areas of life that will be damaged by their perversion that places the need for good stories above all. It leads to a sociopathy inherent in the media dictum of our era "If it bleeds, it leads." This is a sad group of people, not anyone who should be trusted with leadership. They love and promote that which is horrible for the rest of society. They do so, merely because it gives them a story to tell. Corona communism has been good for some journalistic careers, awful for society.

[70] The dishonest – Unfortunately, some people have allowed themselves to be surrounded by liars. Such people are benefitted by knowing the "tells" of the liars around them – those gestures and cues that indicate a change of intent. With a great deal of communication taking place in the face, the dishonest have welcomed mandatory masking as a way to better hide their dishonesty from others. A mask does not belong in what is believed to be a sincere communication. It places the more sincere party at an even greater disadvantage, when all they seek to do is to honestly communicate. This is one of many ways in which mandatory masking feeds a toxic undercurrent in human society. Those who

would deny this may have good reason to want themselves and others masked that go beyond disproven medical claims that these contemporary snake oil salesman are foisting on contemporary society.

[71] The ugly – Mankind has long engaged in ways of appearing more attractive to others. Some people have found a new lease on life during mandatory masking. Concerned about their appearance, unwilling to improve their appearance, they have come to understand that some people don't like the way they look, but may not entirely accept it. There's a certain passive aggression, a dishonesty, toward oneself and others in this lack of acceptance combined with a disinterest in trying. Suddenly in April 2020, a government edict called on all such people to roll out of bed each morning and wear a piece of polypropylene over two thirds of their faces. Two thirds of that ugly thing they've been carrying around their whole lives – that they are unwilling to either accept or alter – is suddenly able to be hidden from the world and doing so is heretofore called "normal." I think many would be surprised to learn how many insecure people like this exist and how secretly happy they are to finally be able to resolve this matter of their mug with little decisiveness on their part.

[72] The dramatic –There are some who like to have a story to tell and others who just want life to, above all, be exciting. There's more to life than titillation, but some leave it at that. Consequently, some really love intrigue, conflict, novelty, and other dramatic happenings in life. They will do all they can to surround themselves with as much drama as possible. For those with a primary love for human individualisms and freedom, the absolute horror of imposing a lockdown on a population, closing the churches, closing businesses, instituting corona communism, and requiring face masks should never again be repeated in human history. To those with a superseding desire for drama, the excitement is just getting started and they can't wait for more. 2020 has provided them with at least twenty years of interesting stories to tell. For people like this, their penchant for the dramatic and their cooperation in the destruction of healthy life should not be underestimated. Entertainment is fantastic. Drama can be a useful tool. Titillation can be enjoyable. Titillation must not be the primary cause for living life.

[73] Maine Department of Economic & Community Development. (2020). Covid-19 Prevention Checklists. Retrieved from https://www.maine.gov/decd/covid-19-prevention-checklists

[74] *The Twilight Zone* was an American television show from the second half of the twentieth century, in which the Kafkaesque and paranormal were often treated as normal. There was a time when the idea of hermetically sealing oneself off from microbes or any other aspect of living life, was seen as a horrible and sad aberration. Movies were made about the sad lives of children who lived in bubbles and day time television might dramatically cover their story. Masks were known for all human time to be a signal of something amiss. A full view of the full human face was natural and comforting and protective to all around. It was an important way you were able to figure out what another person was communicating. A person masked was a person with something to hide. Peace was once a human ideal in order to ensure an orderly and prosperous life.

"Peace is white privilege" was pejoratively chanted on the streets of Portland, Oregon on the night of November 3, 2020. Logic was once seen as part of the highest tool humanity had at its disposal. "Logic is a tool of the patriarchy," is a pejorative rebuttal from some Americans anytime a point too complex is spoken in their presence. 2020 is a Twilight Zone of a year in which that which was once unimaginable has now become so commonplace.

[75] Order of the Health Officer No. C19-12b, California Health and Safety Code § 120295, et seq.; Cal. Penal Code §§ 69, 148(a)(1); San Francisco Administrative Code §7.17(b). (2020).

[76] City and County of San Francisco. (2020). Face coverings protect our entire community from COVID-19. Retrieved from https://sf.gov/information/masks-and-face-coverings-coronavirus-pandemic

[77] Throughout history, doctors have developed names for poorly understood conditions in an effort to maintain the appearance that they know what they are talking about. The most honest doctors engage in no such behavior and willingly say "I'm not sure what happened." or "That isn't well understood by me or anyone I know of." Instead, terms like "consumption," "marasmus," "ague," "catarrh," "nostalgia," and "visitation by God" were once used on death certificates. Sudden Infant Death Syndrome, or SIDS, is a lot like that. We don't know why some children just stop breathing. What we do know, if we are honest with ourselves, is that we barely understand the human body and that breathing is a great mystery to us, providing far more benefit in far more ways than simply the transfer of oxygen and carbon dioxide. Thankfully, because of the great hype and mystery, around SIDS, public health experts are willing to let one group of people – children under 2 – breathe freely across the board. Though the consequences of wearing 10 cent polypropylene masks may not be entirely clear, instinct tells many that children are not the only ones who should live life unmasked and with unrestricted breathing.

[78] Berkowitz, E. (2017). George Bush and the Americans with Disabilities Act. Social Welfare History Project. Retrieved from http://socialwelfare.library. vcu.edu/recollections/george-bush-and-the-americans-with-disabilities-act/

[79] An American president of the late 20th century. Formerly an actor, and fatherly in demeanor, he was effective in encouraging the black and white assessment of the American empire in the world as fundamentally good.

[80] The United States had a bicameral legislature in the 18th, 19th, 20th and 21st centuries, largely dominated by two political parties in a largely bipartisan system. For a period of time the "Democratic Party" was the name of one of those parties.

[81] An American politician of the late 20th century.

[82] An American retailer from the 20th century and first half of the 21st century that sold sundries, popularly categorized as a drug store.

[83] An American retailer from the 20th century and first half of the 21st century that sold sundries, popularly categorized as a drug store.

[84] An American retailer from the 20th century and first half of the 21st century that sold sundries, popularly categorized as a hardware store.

[85] An American retailer from the 20th century and first half of the 21st century that sold sundries, popularly categorized as a hardware store.

[86] An American retailer from the 20th century and first half of the 21st century that sold sundries, popularly categorized as a grocery store.

[87] Farmers markets are a trend from the second half of the 20th century and first half of the 21st century as Western society moved away from the idea that food comes from a farm and started to imagine that food originates in a grocery store, the idea of a farmers market was a popular novelty among some, who rather than changing any of the toxic and anti-human aspects of the thinking that food originates in a grocery store, simply modified their thinking to say "Food originates in a grocery store or a farmers market." Quite satisfied with themselves, it became a mark of virtue among some to express such a concept to their peer group.

[88] Chen, S. (2008). How to play the first bar of Rhapsody in Blue. *The Journal of the Acoustical Society of America*, *123*(5), 3123–3123. Retrieved from https://doi.org/10.1121/1.2933048
"George Gershwin's Rhapsody in Blue opens with a solo clarinet playing a spectacular two-and-a-half octave rise, terminating in a glissando (Figure 1). This first bar of is one of the great icons of 20th century music and one of the best known bars in music. Commissioned by Paul Whiteman and his jazz orchestra, Rhapsody premiered with Gershwin on the piano. It was not until rehearsals of the Rhapsody began that the glissando unintentionally came into being.
> ...as a joke on Gershwin, Gorman (Whiteman's virtuoso clarinetist) played the opening measure with a noticeable glissando, adding what he considered a humorous touch to the passage. Reacting favorably to Gorman's whimsy, Gershwin asked him to perform the opening measure that way at the concert and to add as much of a 'wail' as possible. (Schwartz 1979:81)
At its première on 12 February 1924 at New York's Aeolian Hall, "Ross Gorman began his glissando and electrified the house" (Schiff 1997:60). This performance tradition has continued to delight audiences ever since. Replicating Gorman's 'wail' is now standard practice (Figure 2 is a spectrogram of this feat) but a difficult act to follow. To achieve this effect, expert players combine unusual fingerings with even more unusual configurations of their vocal tract to achieve a nearly continuous rise in playing pitch."

[89] Delta Airlines. (n.d.). Travelers with Disabilities. Retrieved from https://pro.delta.com/content/agency/us/en/products-and-services/special-services/travelerswith-disabilities.html#

[90] Non-Discrimination on the Basis of Disability in Air Travel, 14 CFR Part 382. (2008). Retrieved from https://www.law. cornell.edu/cfr/text/14/part-382

[91] Ferguson, N.M., Laydon, D., Nedjati-Gilani, G., Imai, N., Ainslie, K., Baguelin, M.,...Ghani, A.C. (2020). Report 9: Impact of non-pharmaceutical interventions (NPIs) to reduce COVID-19 mortality and healthcare demand. *Imperial College COVID-19 Response Team.* Retrieved from https://www.imperial.ac.uk/media/imperial-college/medicine/sph/ide/gida-fellowships/Imperial-College-COVID19-NPI-modelling-16-03-2020.pdf

[92] Texas Public Law. (2019). Texas Education Code-Sec. 37.0023 Prohibited Averisve Techniques. Retrieved from https://texas.public.law/statutes/tex._educ._code_section_ 37.0023

[93] Stevo, A.J. (2015). In Poems. CreateSpace Independent Publishing Platform.

[94] Exec. Order No. 2020-153: Masks, *rescission of* Exec. Order No. 2020-147 (2020). Retrieved from https://www.michigan.gov/whitmer/0,9309,7-387-90499_90705-535105--,00.html

[95] Gasnier, L.G. & MacKenzie, D. (Director). (1914). The Perils of Pauline [Film Serial]. General Film Company & Eclectic Film Company.

[96] Akers, B. (2020). Oh, Glorious Promise: "We Will Be Violating the Judge's Order"!!!!. Retrieved from https://www.lewrockwell.com/lrc-blog/oh-glorious-promise-we-will-be-violating-the-judges-order/

[97] Centers for Disease Control and Prevention. (2020). Considerations for Wearing Masks. Retrieved from https://www.cdc.gov/coronavirus/2019-ncov/prevent-getting-sick/cloth-face-cover-guidance.html

[98] Marriott International. (2020). Marriott Mask Exemption Policy. Marriott International News Center. Retrieved from https://news.marriott.com/news/2020/07/20/arne-sorenson-video-update-on-face-coverings

[99] Telford, Taylor. (2020). Marriott, the world's largest hotel chain, will require guests to wear masks in common areas. *The Washington Post.* Retrieved from https://www.washingtonpost.com/travel/2020/07/21/marriott-worlds-largest-hotel-chain-will-require-guests-wear-masks-common-areas/

[100] Oil Sands Magazine. (2017). WTI Specs Get a Minor Makeover in 2018. Retrieved from https://www.oilsandsmagazine.com/news/2017/12/22/west-texas-intermediate-wti-specifications-get-updated-in-2018

[101] Wright, R.E., (2020). Why Aren't Americans Suing Their Way Out of Lockdown?. American Institute for Economic Research. Retrieved from https://www.aier.org/article/why-arent-americans-suing-their-way-out-of-lockdown/

[102] Slings, S.R. (1994). Plato's Apology of Socrates: A Literary and Philosophical Study with a Running Commentary. E.J. Brill.

[103] Centers for Disease Control and Prevention. (2020). How To Protect Yourself. Retrieved from https://www.cdc.gov/coronavirus/2019-ncov/prevent-getting-sick/prevention.html

[104] Centers for Disease Control and Prevention. (2020). Coronavirus Disease 2019 (COVID-19): Know How It Spreads. Retrieved from https://www.cdc.gov/coronavirus/2019-ncov/prevent-getting-sick/prevention.html

[105] Aubrey, A. & Dwyer, C. (2020). CDC Now Recommends Americans Consider Wearing Cloth Face Coverings In Public. NPR News. Retrieved from https://www.npr.org/sections /coronavirus-live-updates/2020/04/03/826219824/president-trump-says-cdc-now-recommends-americans-wear-cloth-masks-in-public

[106] Hansen, C. (2020). CDC Advises All Americans to Wear Cloth Masks in Public. US News. Retrieved from https://www.usnews.com/news/national-news/articles/2020-04-03/cdc-advises-all-americans-to-wear-cloth-masks-in-public

[107] Watson, K. (2020).Trump announces CDC recommends cloth masks in public but says he won't wear one. CBS News. Retrieved from https://www.cbs news.com/news/coronavirus-task-force-update-covid-19-response-watch-live-stream-today-2020-04-03/

[108] Brown, K., Lin II, R., Mergerian, C., Money, L. (2020). CDC recommends wearing face masks during coronavirus pandemic. Los Angeles Times. Retrieved from https://www.latimes.com/science/story/2020-04-03/cdc-recommends-wear ing-face-masks-during-coronavirus-pandemic

[109] Liptak, K. (2020). Trump announces new face mask recommendations after heated internal debate. CNN Politics. Retrieved from https://www.cnn.com/2020/04/03/politics/trump-white-house-face-masks/index.html

[110] Matsakis, A.T. (2014). Loving Someone with PTSD: A Practical Guide to Understanding and Connecting with Your Partner after Trauma (The New Harbinger Loving Someone Series) (1st Edition). New Harbinger Publications. https://www.cnn.com/2020/04/03/politics/trump-white-house-face-masks/index.html

[111] League of Nations – A governmental institution of the first half of the 20th century intended to reduce the amount of self-determination in the hands of the individual. Its stated goal: world peace.
History.com Editors. (2010). League of Nations Instituted. Retrieved from https://www.history.com/this-day-in-history/league-of-nations-instituted

[112] UN – A governmental institution of the second half of the 20th century and the first half of the 21st century intended to reduce the amount of self-determination in the hands of the individual. Its stated purpose: world peace.
United Nations. (n.d.). History of the United Nations. Retrieved from https://www.un.org/en/sections/history/history-united-nations/index.html

[113] Executive Order 6102 – On April 5th, 1933, US president Franklin Delano Roosevelt took it upon himself to decide that Americans no longer had the right to own gold. He also unilaterally determined the price at which that gold would be sold to the government.
Peters, G. & Woolley, J.T. (n.d.). Franklin D. Roosevelt, Executive Order 6102—Requiring Gold Coin, Gold Bullion and Gold Certificates to Be Delivered to the Government Online. The American Presidency Project. Retrieved from https://www.presidency.ucsb.edu/node/208042

[114] Federal Reserve Bank – A governmental institution of the 20th century and the first half of the 21st century intended to reduce the amount of self-determination in the hands of the individual. Its stated goal: greater stability and prosperity.
Board of Governors of the Federal Reserve System. (n.d.). What is the purpose of the Federal Reserve System?. Retrieved from https://www.federalreserve.gov/faqs/about_12594.html
Federal Reserve Bank

[115] Bentley, James. (1984). *Martin Niemöller: 1892–1984*. NY: Macmillan Free Press.

[116] The Society of Gilbert Keith Chesterton. (2012). When Man Cease to Worship God. Retrieved from https://www.chesterton.org/ceases-to-worship/

[117] Swift, J. (2012). Gulliver's Travels Into Several Remote Regions of the World. Benjamin Motte. (Original publication in 1726).

[118] Collman, A. (2020). An Orthodox Jewish community in Brooklyn burned face masks in a bonfire to protest Gov. Cuomo imposing a local coronavirus lockdown on them *Business Insider*. Retrieved from https://www.businessinsider.com/nyc-orthodox-jews-protest-local-lockdown-face-masks-bonfire-2020-10

[119] Stack, L. (2020). Backlash Grows in Orthodox Jewish Areas Over Virus Crackdown by Cuomo. T*he New York Times*. Retrieved from https://www.nytimes.com/2020/10/07/nyregion/orthodox-jews-nyc-coronavirus.html

[120] Hanau, S. (2020). Orthodox Jews in Brooklyn burn masks during massive protest against New York's new COVID rules. Jewish Telegraphic Agency. Retrieved from https://www.jta.org/2020/10/07/health/orthodox-jews-in-brooklyn-burn-masks-during-massive-protest-against-new-yorks-new-covid-restrictions

[121] Shelley - Entropy is normal. Decay is normal. Failure is normal. Abnormal are those who believe they are above that. The epigraph that kicks off the chapter "Why Technocrats Believe In Face Masks" is from the poem "Ozymandias" (1818) by Percy Bysshe Shelley. It appears in its entirety below.

Ozymandias
BY PERCY BYSSHE SHELLEY
I met a traveller from an antique land,
Who said—"Two vast and trunkless legs of stone
Stand in the desert. . . . Near them, on the sand,
Half sunk a shattered visage lies, whose frown,
And wrinkled lip, and sneer of cold command,
Tell that its sculptor well those passions read
Which yet survive, stamped on these lifeless things,
The hand that mocked them, and the heart that fed;
And on the pedestal, these words appear:
My name is Ozymandias, King of Kings;
Look on my Works, ye Mighty, and despair!
Nothing beside remains. Round the decay
Of that colossal Wreck, boundless and bare
The lone and level sands stretch far away."

[122] History.com Editors. (2009). President Eisenhower warns of military-industrial complex. Retrieved from https://www.history.com/this-day-in-history/eisenhower-warns-of-military-industrial-complex

[123] Deviva, J.C., & Zayfert, C. (2011). When Someone You Love Suffers from Posttraumatic Stress: What to Expect and What You Can Do (1st Edition). The Guilford Press.

[124] Centers for Disease Control and Prevention. (2020). Staff. Retrieved from https://wwwnc.cdc.gov/eid/about/staff

[125] Centers for Disease Control and Prevention. (2020). Considerations for Wearing Masks. Retrieved from https://www.cdc.gov/coronavirus/2019-ncov/prevent-getting-sick/cloth-face-cover-guidance.html

[126] Centers for Disease Control and Prevention. (2020). JAMA editorial reviews latest science, while case study shows masks prevented COVID spread. Retrieved from https://www.cdc.gov/media/releases/2020/p0714-americans-to-wear-masks.html

[127] Fong, G. (2020). Nonpharmaceutical Measures for Pandemic Influenza in Nonhealthcare Settings—Social Distancing Measures. *Emerging Infectious Diseases, 26*(5), 976–984. Retrieved from https://doi.org/10.3201/eid2605.190995

[128] Fong, G. (2020). Nonpharmaceutical Measures for Pandemic Influenza in Nonhealthcare Settings—Social Distancing Measures. *Emerging Infectious Diseases, 26*(5), 976–984. Retrieved from https://doi.org/10.3201/eid2605.190995

[129] World Health Organization. (2009). Advice on the use of masks1 in the community setting in Influenza A (H1N1) outbreaks. Retrieved from https://www.who.int/csr/resources/publications/Adviceusemaskscommunityrevised.pdf

[130] Shakespeare, W. (2020). Henry V. Act IV, Scene III, 20-67. Mowat, B.A. & Werstine, P (Eds.). Simon & Schuster. (Original work published 1599).

Index

349

About The Title

About The Title:
An Ode To Henry Hazlitt,
His Life, And Times

Far from attempting to best him with the title or attempting to mimic his greatness, my title is an ode to Henry Hazlitt, to his style, and to the times he lived in. Henry Hazlitt was a brilliant thinker of economics in his life and through his 1946 book, *Economics in One Lesson,* which became a classic.

He writes a lesson and then applies that lesson, a fantastic rhetorical and pedagogical technique. I attempt to do the same.

Lots of parts of life rhyme and repeat once you start to understand some of the basic concepts by which life operates.

Truth, wisdom, philosophy, religion are all ideas people use to try to tap into the rules of life.

Hazlitt had no monopoly on the truth, he was simply an observer with a scientific way of thinking. In fact he authored another book, which I am a fan of, *The Science of Thinking.*

He was one who thought critically and shared his findings willingly.

As such, he fit perfectly in a role he had at America's Gray Lady, the newspaper of record. In 1946, the US had just completed a war said to be against fascism and extraterritorial aggression, lead by the socialist FDR and by many with extraterritorial ambitions. Those causes for war certainly weren't the most intellectually consistent ones.

Curiously, quite a few Americans returned from the war, seeking to build an America that looked a lot more like something Stalinist, Hitlerian, or Trotskyist and a lot less like the America envisioned in 1776, in Jefferson's third draft of *The Declaration of Independence.*

That was the intellectually consistent draft, where the young firebrand freed the slaves, an idea that lasted mere hours before unsuccessfully making its way through committee.

America today can be accurately described as fascist, socialist, even Marxist. The collectivist and communitarian spirit rules the day in so many regards.

This "long march through the institutions" that collectivists promised, is finally bearing fruit. 2020 has been a most miserable year for so many, because it is the first year America has fully found itself led by those communitarians and collectivists that so occupy the technocratic class of the West.

In 1946, Henry Hazlitt, as he wrote his classic *Economics in One Lesson* served on the editorial board of *The New York Times*.

It was a different time. To even suggest the free market in the halls of the glass house of *The New York Times* on 41th Street in midtown Manhattan is to write your own pink slip.

Meritocracy may have unequal outcomes when measured across demographics that seek to make people a mere member of a group rather than an individual and therefore curiously, support of meritocracy and praise for individual achievement, is claimed to be support of the most ugly racial, gender, and class biases possible.

To suggest logic, reason, and evidence is to prove your own privilege as a member of the patriarchy. For "logic is a tool of the patriarchy."

To aspire to excellence is to do so out of bias, for "excellence is white privilege."

We are a far cry from an era in which all Americans could take some pride in the journalism taking place at *The New York Times* and to be able to find value in its nationally circulated Sunday papers.

In fact, one of America's brightest civil libertarians – Glen Greenwald – created a new media competitor to *The New*

York Times, only dedicated to telling the truth. On October 29, 2020 he was forced out of his own news organization for telling too much truth about American politicians.

We are a far cry from an America that could have a thinker the likes of Henry Hazlitt writing in the editorial pages of *The New York Times* as he did for twelve years from 1934 to 1946 on the topic of economics both signed and unsigned columns.

Yet, that vision of America may forever be lost. In a remnant of people who I know, interact with, and have come to respect and hold in the highest regard – an even better version of America is upheld and in its infancy.

It's a renewed American experiment, Western experiment, classical liberal experiment, free market experiment.

Walking the streets of this country in every corner from the streets of Idaho to the the streets of San Francisco, are members of the quiet, relatively small, remnant, not just keeping the torch burning, but who are actively spreading brushfires of liberty in the minds of men.

I have never lived in darker days than 2020, for the tyranny is so great on the globe and it is led by Americans and the mass of Americans who so support it.

Under American leadership and the majority consent of the governed, America is set to become worse than anything created by Hitler, Stalin, or Mao and how unsurprising it is that the totalitarians of the last century have such support in the political halls of DC, the financial halls of New York City, and in state capitals and counties and cities across this land.

Dark days indeed, if it weren't for the remnant I see, more brightly, more actively than they have ever been my entire life.

A great philosophical battle is ahead. I don't know how it will end. I know we are in the middle of it and I know it is the greatest epic ever written, that I am seeing unfold before me.

I cannot overstate what a joy it has been and will continue to be to engage in that battle.

With the cocky assurance that my ideas are more just, that I know who Darth Vader is, that I know where the Death Star is, that I can see steps ahead with the clarity of mind and spirit I've been given the chance to develop, I know such a beautiful battle lays ahead.

And I cannot imagine better people to walk alongside.

A wordsmith[130] of the highest caliber once commented on the joys of fighting a fight in the minority, the passionate minority. The smaller the number, the greater the honor.

On December 7, 2007, the first Tea Party event of the contemporary Tea Party movement was held in Strasbourg, France. On that day we read there, outside the European Parliament, a piece of writing from that wordsmith as inspiring today and, as fitting as it was then.

If we are mark'd to die, we are enough
To do our country loss; and if to live,
The fewer men, the greater share of honour.
God's will! I pray thee, wish not one man more.
By Jove, I am not covetous for gold,
Nor care I who doth feed upon my cost;
It yearns me not
if men my garments wear;
Such outward things dwell not in my desires:
But if it be a sin to covet honour,
I am the most offending soul alive.
No, faith, my coz, wish not a man from England:
God's peace! I would not lose so great an honour
As one man more, methinks, would share from me
For the best hope I have. O, do not wish one more!
Rather proclaim it, Westmoreland, through my host,
That he which hath no stomach to this fight,
Let him depart; his passport shall be made
And crowns for convoy put into his purse
We would not die in that man's company
That fears his fellowship to die with us.
This day is called the feast of Crispian:
He that outlives this day, and comes safe home,

Will stand a tip-toe when the day is named,
And rouse him at the name of Crispian.
He that shall live this day, and see old age,
Will yearly on the vigil feast his neighbours,
And say 'To-morrow is Saint Crispian:'
Then will he strip his sleeve and show his scars.
And say 'These wounds I had on Crispin's day.'
Old men forget: yet all shall be forgot,
But he'll remember with advantages
What feats he did that day: then shall our names,
Familiar in his mouth as household words,
Harry the king, Bedford and Exeter,
Warwick and Talbot, Salisbury and Gloucester,
Be in their flowing cups freshly remember'd.
This story shall the good man teach his son;
And Crispin Crispian shall ne'er go by,
From this day to the ending of the world,
But we in it shall be remember'd;
We few, we happy few, we band of brothers;
For he to-day that sheds his blood with me
Shall be my brother; be he ne'er so vile,
This day shall gentle his condition:
And gentlemen in England now a-bed
Shall think themselves accursed they were not here,
And hold their manhoods cheap whiles any speaks
That fought with us upon Saint Crispin's day.

Will you join me?

About The Author

About The Author

Allan Stevo has been a tireless advocate for more fair treatment of individuals under the law for over two decades. From the disabled to those with severe medical conditions, Stevo has pushed for individualized approaches, rather than the one-size-fits-all treatment our institution often foists upon those most in need. *Face Masks in One Lesson* demonstrates how and why that individualized, patient-centric approach must be continued for the benefit of those most in need.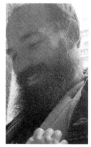

He has spoken to audiences at the University of Chicago, MIT, and dozens of other top schools in the US and around the world. In 2012, he became a best selling author and in 2014, a syndicated columnist.

His writing has appeared widely in publications as diverse as: *The Hill, Roll Call, The Daily Caller, Economic Policy Journal, LewRockwell.com, The Tenth Amendment Center,* and *The Daily Bell.*

In print publications such as *The New York Post, Cleveland Plain Dealer, Buffalo News, Anchorage Press, Lexington Leader, Epoch Times, Nevada Legal Review,* and at think-tanks such as the Manhattan Institute's *City Journal, The Cobden Center, Mises.org,* and many others.

His work has been written about and featured on *CNN, Huffington Post, Bloomberg, New York Times, Wall Street Journal, Reuter's,* and the *Chicago Tribune.*

Stevo's influential writing has been described as "a precedence of sanity," "the truth in print," and "a beacon of liberty." Stevo's been described as "one of the rare individuals who operate under reason and logic." Reading *Face Masks in One Lesson* "might be the most important thing you can do for yourself, your family, and your country," writes Professor Robert Wright.

"What does Stevo's writing mean to me?" asks Dr. Walter Block "All the world."

Face Masks in One Lesson provides the ultimate response to mandatory masking, and is an irreplaceable tool for those who will not go masked another day.

Printed in Great Britain
by Amazon

54957641R00232